Mental Health Issu
the Media

An introduction for health professionals

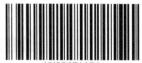

Gary Morris

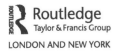

Routledge
Taylor & Francis Group

LONDON AND NEW YORK

First published 2006 by Routledge
2 Park Square, Milton Park, Abingdon, Oxon OX14 4RN

Simultaneously published in the USA and Canada
by Routledge
711 Third Ave, New York, NY 10017

Routledge is an imprint of the Taylor & Francis Group, an informa business

© 2006 Gary Morris

Typeset in Times by
RefineCatch Limited, Bungay, Suffolk

British Library Cataloguing in Publication Data
A catalogue record for this book is available from the British Library

Library of Congress Cataloging in Publication Data
Morris, Gary, 1962–
  Mental health issues and the media : an introduction for health
professionals / Gary Morris.
    p. ; cm.
  Includes bibliographical references and index.
  1. Mental health.   2. Mass media in mental health education.
3. Health in mass media.   I. Title.
  [DNLM: 1. Communications Media.   2. Mental Health.   3. Health
Knowledge, Attitudes, Practices.   WM 105 M876m   2006]
RA790.53.M67   2006
                                    362.2—dc22   2005023846

ISBN10: 0–415–32530–7 (hbk)
ISBN10: 0–415–32531–5 (pbk)
ISBN10: 0–203–358228 (ebk)

ISBN13: 978–0–415–32530–1 (hbk)
ISBN13: 978–0–415–32531–8 (pbk)
ISBN13: 978–0–203–35822–1 (ebk)

Mental Health Issues and the Media

Our ideas about mental health and illness can be informed by personal experiences but are most often formed by the prevailing attitudes of society. A wide range of contemporary media helps create these attitudes and for all health professionals the ways in which they do so are of immediate concern. Health professionals need to:

- be aware of media influences on their own perceptions and attitudes
- take account of both the negative and positive aspects of media intervention in mental health promotion and public education
- understand the way in which we all interact with media messages and how this affects both practitioners and service-users

Mental Health Issues and the Media provides students and professionals in nursing and allied professions, psychiatry, psychology and related disciplines, with a theoretically grounded introduction to the ways in which our attitudes are shaped by the media. Covering the press, literature, film, television and the Internet, it also includes practical advice and recommendations on how to combat negative images for service-users, health care workers and media personnel.

Gary Morris is a Mental Health Nursing Lecturer working at the University of Leeds, UK, where he runs, amongst other courses, a taught module entitled 'Mental Health Issues and the Media'.

To
Lottie, William, Sam,
Daisy and Caitlin

Contents

Figures

Acknowledgements

I would like to acknowledge the support and assistance I have received from a number of people whose help has been vital to the process of writing this book.

First, I owe an immeasurable sense of gratitude to my wife Emily for her tireless support and insightful advice at every stage of this process. This has enabled me to maintain my levels of energy and enthusiasm as well as my focus for this work especially at times when it felt a struggle.

A massive thank you has to be extended to my colleague, Jack Morris, for his collaboration throughout, both in the development as well as the running of the taught module 'Mental Health Issues and the Media'. This has provided the impetus for this publication. This module has been offered on numerous occasions at the University of Leeds and has attracted an extremely wide number and eclectic range of students. Many of the issues addressed within this book are inspired directly through our frequent discussions and planning meetings concerning themes and frameworks for inclusion. It is clear to say that without the valuable support and experience that he has brought to this entire project, none of it would have progressed further than the initial contemplation stage.

I would also like to acknowledge the much-needed and experienced contributions I have received from Pauline Bispham, Marie Clough, Anna Davie, Ian Harrow, Steve Howarth and Peter Morrall. Their thought-provoking and stimulating contributions have provided me with fresh and inspired perspectives from which to revisit material.

I must also mention the excellent and supportive feedback received from the Taylor & Francis team throughout this project who notably include Stephanie Kerrigan, Amanda Lastoria, Margaret Lipscomb, Kirsty Smy and Edwina Wellham.

Finally, many thanks to all the students on the taught module for their invaluable assistance and challenging engagement with some of the themes developed within this publication.

1 The mental health–media relationship

What is this book about?

This book is primarily about a relationship. It addresses the ways in which we as individuals and collectively as a society interact with mental health issues and the extent to which this relationship is changed as a result of media exposure. What we know or how we feel about those who are categorised or labelled as 'mentally ill' is subject to continual change and is influenced by the type of information accessed and the degree of credibility afforded its source. The range of messages that carry mental health themes is vast and we are exposed on a daily basis to a plethora of themes through an ever-increasing selection of media. All of this plays a significant part in the construction of what we know or what we feel about issues connected with the topic of mental health and our ways of relating which may either be of a connecting or distancing type. This relates to the degree to which we are able either to connect with and get closer to understanding the inner world of those affected by mental health problems or to maintain a 'safe' but uninformed distance.

The first element of this relationship concerns what we know. Much of what we learn about the world around us comes from messages transmitted by the wide selection of media types available. We are literally bombarded with segments of information from the moment we wake until the time of finally retiring to bed. On a typical day this might include trawling through the paper, watching television, listening to the radio, visiting Internet sites, watching a film and reading a book as perhaps the more obvious means. We also engage with other media messages from formats such as advertising, stage production, the music industry and the world of art. All of these examples have multiple sub-divisions or genres that further widen the scope and variety of what is on offer. Ongoing advancements within telecommunications and digital television bring fresh new sources to add to this selection. It is important also to consider what is learnt indirectly or second-hand from others who have been exposed to media messages. The chain of communication can be extended to create a form of Chinese whispers with the authority of information being diminished with each successive link. It is hardly surprising therefore that our understanding of mental health issues can end up wildly inaccurate or that it might prove difficult and confusing trying to discriminate between the various sources from which our knowledge originates.

These issues are all explored in detail throughout this book that is essentially (as Figure 1.1 illustrates) about a relationship. This namely concerns a tripartite relationship between: a) us as *individuals* (or collectively as a *society*); b) *mental health issues*; and c) the *media*. It addresses and examines the myriad of processes that play a part in this relationship and how all of those involved exert a degree of influence over the others. Each participant shares some of the overall responsibility as to the outcome of this relationship as we can, for example, place the blame upon the tabloid press for biased and insensitive reporting although disregard the fact that we as a society are aiding and encouraging this process by continuing to buy their products. Clearly, each of those involved has a distinctly different perspective and separate interests that influence the way in which they relate to certain aspects. It is the significance of these factors and the impact upon the overall relationship that forms the main focus addressed within this book.

In order to begin exploring these themes, it is important to look in detail at each of the following participants within this tripartite relationship: individuals/society; mental health issues; and the media.

Individuals/society

Definitions of the term *society* include:

> 'The institutions and culture of a distinct self-perpetuating group.'
> 'The totality of social relationships among humans.'
>
> (Dictionary.com 2005)

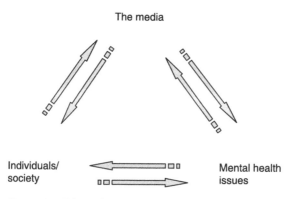

Figure 1.1 Tri-partite relationship.

'The fact or condition of being connected or related.'
(*Oxford English Dictionary* 2005)

What emerges strongly from these definitions is that *society* is primarily concerned with a set of relationships between its members with regard to what is shared. The term *society* can be regarded as a collective entity or broken down into separate components containing *individuals* or groupings of individuals. The Gestalt focus upon 'the whole' being more than the sum of its parts (Köhler 1947) fits very aptly here in that individuals in society should be seen not simply in fractional terms but as dynamic and influential components whose identity is formed through their interaction and relationships with others in 'the whole'. There are numerous sub-groupings or sets each representing differing values or beliefs. As individuals we naturally belong to a number of these sub-groups each of which has its own collective viewpoints and influences. The family provides us with our first significant group experience and is followed by others such as those encountered through schooling, leisure activities, religion, employment, political affiliation, health care and a potentially endless list of many others.

Individuals hold multiple roles, their relationships being governed by the different sub-groups to which they belong (Epting 1984). Within different contexts what is expected of us, how we perceive ourselves and how we respond will naturally vary. Within the family, for example, as a parent or partner we may have significantly different ways of interacting with others than we do at work with colleagues and employers. We are constantly modifying our thoughts, attitudes and behaviours in response to the accompanying feedback and reinforcers we are exposed to. This can be related to concepts such as social identity or personal identity as identified by Gripsrud (2002). The former relates to what we get from others' perceptions of us and the shared contexts that we are part of (e.g. culture, gender) and the personal identity being what makes us unique and distinguishable from others.

The component *individual/society* can therefore be regarded as a dynamic and multifaceted entity either regarded as a number of distinct and unique individuals, a varied set of sub-groupings or as a collective whole. The qualities and values held by this component therefore depend heavily upon specific experience and the range of pressures and influences which individuals or groups are exposed to.

Mental health issues

The term *mental health issues* is a vastly encompassing one having many different attributable meanings. We can consider the actual words themselves, which evoke wildly differing associations and interpretations. The strongest and most impactful of the three words here is undoubtedly that of '*mental*'. It is a word which, depending upon the context of its use, may have either positive or negative connotations. On the favourable side, the word *mental* can be related to aspects such as *cerebral*, which denotes enhanced cognitive ability. This word may therefore evoke thoughts of individuals such as Einstein or Newton and signify qualities such as high levels of intelligence. These are esteemed and valued connections that afford a true sense of value and worth to whomever they are applied. At the opposite end of the spectrum is a far from flattering association. It is where the word *mental* is used as a form of derision, something that greatly undermines and reduces the credibility of the individual it is applied to. It is often used dismissively and seemingly unconcerned about a person's felt experience. When appearing in newspaper headlines it can drastically influence the impression given – for example, the *Daily Express*'s 'Bruno Put in *Mental* Home', or on another occasion, the *Independent*'s '*Mental* Patient Freed to Kill'. The use of words in this manner is commonly found within many media products and serves to reinforce negative attitudes held by the general public.

The wider term *mental health issues* can be looked at in two contrasting ways but is perhaps more commonly associated with that of *mental illness* over that of *mental well-being*. The former term carries a number of stereotypical associations including the exaggerated propensity for violence. This highlights a commonly held fear that those with mental health problems are unpredictable and more prone to aggressive acts than other members of the population (Morrall 2000a). Other negative connotations include the underlying assumption that the 'mentally ill' are unable to adequately care for themselves (Health Education Authority 1999). This brings about a pitying and disempowering approach, which diminishes an individual's sense of autonomy or choice. By contrast, the less applied connotation of *mental well-being* is associated with aspects such as campaigning and health promotion initiatives.

Another association is that of *mental health treatment*, something generally viewed with a sense of trepidation and fear, borne out of striking and lasting images seen in media examples such as in the film *One Flew over the Cuckoo's Nest* (Seale 2002). This type of portrayal is made more frightening by the strong sense of powerlessness attributed to those receiving care. Examples such as these reflect the destructive culture of institutionalised care outlined in some depth a few decades ago by the social researchers Goffman (1961) and Barton (1976). Clearly, many people's understanding of treatment is inaccurately fuelled by various impactful sources that do not properly convey the range and scope of current care approaches available. Fortunately there do exist within the media a variety of examples showing treatment as a caring process as evidenced in the films *Good Will Hunting* and *Ordinary People* that portray the helpful and enabling side of mental health care.

To conclude this section, another issue worthy of mention is the term *mental health legislation*. This covers a largely polarised set of opinions with, at one end of the spectrum, feelings that not enough control is being taken with unsupervised and 'unwell' individuals being left to roam the streets. At the other end, the proposals for added levels of constraint are viewed with some concern, particularly with worries about the ways in which this might further breach and impinge upon an individuals' freedom. Proposed governmental changes in the Draft Mental Health Bill (Department of Health (DOH) 2004) enables people to be detained in hospital and given treatment against their will. While this is welcomed in some quarters in others it is greeted with suspicion and distrust. In particular, comments by the mental health charity Mind (2004a) express concerns regarding the wide range of people and types of treatment included within this new legislation providing for compulsory treatment and loss of liberty. The main argument being raised by mental health advocates concerns the availability of effective treatment and support over that of detention and exclusion (Mental Health Media 2004; Mind 2004a)

The media

The term *media* can be understood simply as a means of communication by organisations or individuals with a targeted audience. Messages are transmitted via a number of communicating channels and are interacted upon by a receiver primarily through the senses of sight and sound. Information is inputted in forms such as narrative (either printed or spoken), imagery (light, colour, appearance, expressions and gestures) or as sound (music and verbal exclamations).

A number of distinctions are made with regards to the term *media* including those of *mass media* and *new media*. The mass media may be understood simply as a communicating agent that can reach potentially large numbers of people in a diverse range of social settings (Devereux 2003). The concept here of wide reach is supported by McQuail (2005), who indicates the ability the *mass media* has in acting as a cohesive force connecting scattered individuals in a shared experience. This picture is changing with the advent of *new media* as the concept of an audience as a mass entity is becoming more fragmented in light of the greater number of media providers and products available. We can understand the term *new media* with regards to the recent technological developments within telecommunications that notably include the Internet and digital television services (Stevenson 2002).

The *media* itself is a communicating entity that has provided its audiences with forms of entertainment and education for many centuries. Historically this involved traditional forms such as art, writing and drama. The range of media types available changed rapidly especially with advancements in scientific and technological endeavours from the late nineteenth century onwards. There was a greater accessibility to the written word through the development of the printing press by William Caxton in 1477, commencing with the publication a year later of *Dictes or Sayengis of the Philosophres*. Nowadays, an almost limitless array of newspapers, magazines and books are published, geared towards every conceivable format or interest group.

The era of photography began with the announcement on 7 January 1839 of the development of the Daguerreotype, the first successful photographic process. The process consisted of exposing copper plates to iodine, the fumes forming a light-sensitive silver iodide. This led on to the search for animated or moving pictures with early inventions including the 'wheel of life' or the 'zoopraxiscope', where moving drawings or photographs were watched through a slit in the side. Modern motion picture making began with the invention of the motion picture camera in 1895, largely credited to the Frenchman Louis Lumière. Three decades later, *The Jazz Singer*, made in 1927, was the first feature length film to use recorded song and dialogue.

The birth of radio dates back to 1885 when Marconi sent and received his first radio signal. In 1924, John Logie Baird demonstrated a television system which transmitted an outline of objects and followed this a year later with an improved system which showed the head of a dummy as a real image. These achievements have continued to develop at a rapid pace with a virtual explosion in the number of channels now offered through cable and satellite services. This has been followed with the advent of digital television and radio services.

This brings us on to new media and in particular the birth of the Internet, whose origins date back to the 1960s with the development of a technology where strings of data were broken down and reassembled at their destination (LaBruzza 1997). This is complemented by further advances in telecommunication technology heralding an era of greater interactivity between the sender and receiver. The huge selection of media products now available does allow for much greater consumer choice although it poses problems with regard to examining the concept of audience reception because of the scale and complexity of the possible channels and sources involved (McQuail 1992).

Relationships

Having looked briefly at each of the participants in turn we can now focus our attention upon the relationship they have with each other leading towards an appreciation of the total relationship.

Society's relationship with mental health

This is an exceedingly complex relationship to describe and perhaps is better understood not by a single relationship but a set of multifaceted ones. Within society, there are many different ways in which mental health issues are encountered. Contact may be close or distant, informed or misinformed, personal or professional. We understand and react to those experiencing mental health problems as a consequence of what we know and what we feel. A core consideration regarding this relationship relates to *who* within the perspective of *society* is being considered. The following categorisations provide a useful means of exploring the very diverse range of vantage points involved: personal experience; professional experience; *victims* of the mentally ill; the mentally ill as *victims*; and the inexperienced.

Personal experience

Personal experience of mental health problems might incorporate either one's own direct experience as a mental health service-user or as a carer to family and friends. This potentially will predispose those involved to being more informed and sensitive towards mental health issues than those without an appreciation of the actual reality of these experiences. Recognition of this leads to those with a direct understanding of the actual lived experience of mental health problems being afforded a greater sense of authority and credibility. This has led individuals and organisations such as Mind and Rethink to become actively involved in mental health campaigning and in providing a range of services, resources and support networks.

The nature of a person's experience and the eventual outcome will naturally have a significant impact upon how mental health issues are regarded. For instance, we can consider a range of experiences falling somewhere along a continuum from destructiveness at one pole towards survival at the other. People who have received good, supportive care and have been able to work through their problems and rebuild their lives will clearly have a different perspective than those who are, for example, actively depressed and feeling let down by agencies of care. The wide range of differing perspectives here can be verified through reviewing sources such as personal Internet sites which provide well-informed, helpful and informative sites alongside those that are overly subjective, wildly inaccurate and harmful.

Professional experience

For the purpose of this category, professional experience can be taken to incorporate not only those on a professional register but all the allied health care support personnel as well. Those involved in professional caring roles will have their own thoughts and feelings concerning those with mental health problems. Naturally there will in a number of cases be an overlap between this and the previous group where individuals have both a professional and personal experience of mental health issues. The nature of a person's clinical experience and the philosophy and approaches to care encountered is important. For example, some nursing homes caring for people with dementia utilise approaches to care reflecting a culture of paternalism believing that clients are to be 'looked after' and that carers know best what their needs might be. While in a number of instances representing well-meaning approaches to care, this approach, as highlighted by the work of Tom Kitwood and the Bradford Dementia Group, reduces personal choice and freedom and has a detrimental effect upon those concerned (Kitwood 1997). This opinion originates in some of the widely held stereotypes such as the view that people with mental health problems are unable to care for themselves sufficiently. It is sharply contrasted by clinical approaches that demonstrate a greater focus upon family involvement, client-centred work and collaborative working relationships as advocated by a number of writers within the person-centred domain (Rogers 1961; Peplau 1988).

Victims of the 'mentally ill'

The descriptor here should be widened to encompass all those who feel themselves to be victims of those who are regarded as mentally ill irrespective of what the reality of the situation actually is. Obviously we have individuals who are clearly affected in tragic ways such as Jane Zito whose husband Jonathan was killed in a London tube station by Christopher Clunis, a man diagnosed with schizophrenia and with a long history of violence, institutional care and non-compliance with treatment programmes (Zito Trust 2005). We may also include other individuals here who have felt intimidated or uncomfortable regardless of the actual level of threat they have been exposed to. The reason for this is because of the way in which they feel about the mentally ill and any resultant response can be engendered irrespective of how others might regard or frame the same situation. Therefore the word *victim* can range from actual experience of physical or verbal abuse through to a feeling of insecurity or discomfort engendered by those with mental health problems. One of the core aspects here relates to how felt or perceived experience influences one's subsequent thoughts and behaviour. A useful frame of reference here is O'Connor and Seymour's (1990) model (see Figure 1.2) which addresses the relationship between feelings and behaviour.

The essence of this model is that of interaction where the behaviour of one person generates an internal feeling in the other which in turn influences their subsequent behaviour. For example, Person A is admitted to a mental health unit and feels lost, intimidated and frightened (*internal response*). He behaves

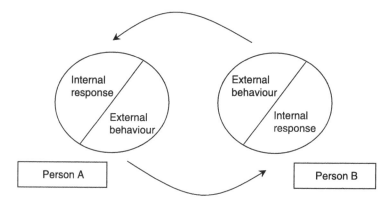

Figure 1.2 Internal response and external behaviour. Adapted from O'Connor and Seymour (1990).

by questioning and challenging staff in a somewhat forceful manner attempting to regain some feeling of control (*external behaviour*). This is interpreted as aggressive and intimidating by the health care professional (Person B), who feels threatened and uncertain (*internal response*). She reacts defensively and attempts to assert herself by outlining, rather more forcefully than necessary, the unit protocols regarding aggressive behaviour (*external behaviour*). This in turn reinforces the intimidated feelings of the client and the dynamic illustrated here continues to progress in a somewhat negative spiral.

The essence then of this category is of individuals who predominately feel either intimidated or antagonistic towards those with mental health problems. Their fears and lack of security are heightened and reinforced through continued media coverage of the negative kind where stigmatising and ill-informed portrayals can be found in abundance. It covers in particular the proliferation of media examples where mental health issues are associated with a sense of violence or dangerousness (Morrall 2000a).

The mentally ill as victims

This category includes those with mental health problems who perceive themselves in the role of victims. As with the previous category, the emphasis here is on a felt or perceived experience that may differ significantly from what is actually encountered. There are a number of negative reinforcements which help to shape this perception such as incidences of rejection and alienation felt from the general public; a relegation of roles or one's position within the family; or an abusive or disempowering experience of health care. As illustrated by Skinner (1974), an individual's behaviour is shaped and maintained by consequences as what happens afterwards will determine whether or not it will be repeated (being strengthened) or will stop (becoming weakened). As individuals with mental health problems fall into one of the main groups in society who encounter stigma (Bloch and Singh 1997) – and there are countless examples throughout history of them being badly treated and socially excluded (Wing 1978) – the feelings of victimisation are exacerbated. It is also heightened by the continued use of jargonistic and abusive terminology (e.g. 'loonies', 'psycho' or 'mentals') that has been freely used both within society and the media in what may be either a thoughtless or intentful manner (Wahl 1995; Philo 1996a).

The negative impact upon those with mental health problems who consider themselves to be *victims* either of a health care system or by their communities cannot be underestimated. This can be seen through Cooley's '*The looking glass self*' whereby a person's identity and self-concept is built primarily as a result of how others act and respond towards them (Cohen 1982). The impact of disempowering and rejecting approaches therefore by others can leave individuals within this category feeling marginalised, rejected and helpless. As Mind's (2000) *Counting the Cost* report highlights, negative public attitudes and stigmatising media portrayals serve to enhance a person's feeling of isolation and lowered self-esteem. They are also subsequently less motivated towards seeking support because of the stigma surrounding mental health care.

The inexperienced (general or lay public)

This category includes those with little direct involvement or experience. The majority of what people within this grouping know about mental health issues is gathered second-hand, namely what has been related by others or extrapolated from the media. In a sense this might also include those with mental health problems as experience of any one specific mental health state does not necessarily mean that individuals will be more tuned into the experience of others. For instance, people suffering with depression or anxiety have a completely separate concept of what mental illness means when compared, for example, to the experience of altered cognition and delusional thought patterns encountered with schizophrenia. Finer distinctions may even be made within single mental health conditions as, for example, one person's experience of bereavement will be uniquely different to that of others. This is affected by factors such as the type of relationship held with the deceased (e.g. one of dependency) and the subsequent impact this has upon their role. Each person therefore has their own unique and distinctive experience and understanding as to what the term mental illness actually means. What needs recognising is the vast spectrum of difference encompassed within the term 'mental illness' instead of seeing everyone concerned as belonging to one collective 'mass' upon whom we attribute similar qualities, for example, potentially violent, 'mad', or unpredictable. Another aspect worthy of mention is the degree of hierarchy that exists with regard to mental health problems as distinctions and gradings are made between certain conditions. If looking for instance at the classifications of neuroses and psychoses, it is the former which tends to be perceived in general more sympathetically compared to the latter which is seen less favourably and with a greater degree of stigma being applied. This is evidenced clearly within newspaper headlines that treat conditions such as depression (e.g. 'Sad Kerry' – *The Sun*) very differently from those that fall within the category of psychoses where fear and mistrust are strongly reflected (e.g. 'I ate his brains . . . lovely' – *Daily Mirror*). The psychotic classification clearly lends itself to a more dramatic portrayal reflected in, although helping to build up, an inaccurate and unbalanced view among the general public. This creates the dichotomy which exists for some whereby some types of mental health problems are to be pitied whereas others are to be feared.

Misinformation and stereotypes can be so pervasive and powerful that we accept certain elements without question as representing the truth. In terms of collective learning, it is hard to separate out what has been learnt from credible and reliable sources and what has been obtained from other less reliable ones. We may feel so certain about particular issues (e.g. the danger potential of those with mental health problems) that we are not swayed even when in possession of fuller and more accurate facts. This can be illustrated by reflecting back in time to an era when the certainty and belief that the world was flat led to much anxiety when setting sail in search of new lands. This erroneous belief was supported at the time by a good deal of 'reliable' evidence until being clearly disproved a number of years later. The way in which the mentally ill are viewed has changed enormously over the years and the concept of 'insanity' has been regarded as many things including an excess of bodily humours; an indication of moral weakness; demonic possession; a sign of witchcraft; a sense of feebleness; a response to environmental factors; or, as indicated by Thomas Szasz (1992) and R.D. Laing (1990), an experience which exists as a social construction. What is evident though is that despite the ever-changing connotations of the term mental illness, negative feelings and associations continue to proliferate in our thinking and treatment towards those concerned.

Society's relationship with the media

The relationship between society and the media can be regarded on a cyclical basis with each participant in turn exerting a sense of influence upon the other (see Figure 1.3). There is wide-ranging debate as to which is the more powerful agent within this relationship; societal attitudes or media depictions. One element, subject to much study over the years, relates to the impact that media exposure has upon people's subsequent attitude and behaviour. The prevailing view is that the mass media has a degree of power in effecting social change through the distribution among a population of opinion, beliefs, values and practices (McQuail 2005). A focus for many studies has been that of 'media effects' and the work of individuals such as Albert Bandura (1986) on social learning theory. This approach details the direct influence that exposure to modelled behaviour has and relates to aspects such as the reported increases in suicide attempts following scenes depicted in television dramas (Hawton *et al.* 1999). The media effects model has, though, been greeted with a fair degree of criticism over recent years because of the overly simplistic manner in which it has been applied and the lack of attention to various aspects whereby audience members are able to respond differently to media examples or come up with their own interpretations (Gauntlett 1995). It is interesting therefore to note Noble's (1973) findings which demonstrated that 6-year-old children exposed to violence on television discriminated

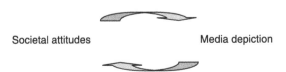

Societal attitudes   Media depiction

Figure 1.3 Societal attitudes and media depiction relationship.

between the different styles of production they were exposed to. Documentaries and more realistic scenes made them anxious whereas the more stylised and distanced scenes of violence proved stimulating regarding their play. Another view is that in some cases it might be cathartic to have some exposure to violent portrayals as evidenced by Feshbach and Singer's (1971) study whereby it was found that watching programmes with a violent content for some participants helped to control aggression by purifying them of such impulses. While acknowledging that media effects do not address the whole picture, there is no question that they do have some effect. While claims might be made by tobacco companies to the effect that the power of tobacco advertising does not directly encourage the uptake of smoking but merely influences brand choice, it is hard then to understand the huge increase in smoking in third world countries noted by organisations such as Action on Smoking and Health (ASH 2005) following major and sustained marketing campaigns. Likewise, many media professionals reject the notion that they are responsible for the perpetuation of harmful stereotypes, claiming that they merely mirror the values and beliefs of society (Bolton 2000). Whether we accept this statement or not there is certainly some strong evidence to suggest that stigmatising media coverage does have a detrimental effect upon creating the stereotypical and negative beliefs which are then being 'mirrored'. The core issue here is to do with responsibility and accountability for some of the destructive content being relayed by media groups and it is not acceptable to simply deflect criticism elsewhere. There is an appetite among the public for dramatic and sensational coverage as evidenced through ratings, box office receipts and sales circulation, but it is irresponsible to simply meet this need and perpetuate the debilitating impact this has upon those with mental health problems (Mind 2000). Although there are instances when drivers slow down through curiosity to look at a car crash it would clearly be tasteless to produce videos of real-life accidents to meet this perceived need. Likewise, media providers should be held to account for the output of insensitive and inaccurate material regarding mental health issues that continues to be produced in direct contravention of their own regulatory standards.

Conversely, the media are in a sense reflecting what are the current views and beliefs concerning mental illness. This is shown very clearly through historical examples where the type of portrayal reflects the thinking of that era. The range of variations of depiction concerning the term madness is vast and, as stated by Wing:

> Madness can stand for every variety of unreason from foolery to psychosis . . . [and] carries different meanings according to the epoch, the society, and the social group involved, and according to the interests and preconceptions of the person who is using it.

(Wing 1978: 2)

Ancient views about madness predominantly had divine connotations with explanations of it being a punishment visited upon humankind by the gods (Porter 2002). An example can be found in the Old Testament (Deuteronomy 6: 5) which relates how Nebuchadnezzar is punished by God with the line 'the lord will smite thee with madness'. Early Greek attitudes towards mental health were derived from myths and epics. These again had divine connotations such as the visitation upon Heracles by the gods of a force which heralded his period of madness. We can also look at eighteenth and nineteenth-century literature and the reflection of generally held assumptions that madness was regarded as an extension of the female condition (Small 1996). The era of incarceration is well-represented by portrayals such as Hogarth's *Rake's Progress*, the films *Asylum* and *Bedlam*, and Ken Kesey's seminal *One Flew over the Cuckoo's Nest*, all of which powerfully reflected the thinking of their day. It is therefore not surprising with the advent of Community Care (following the Community Care Act (DOH 1990)) to find a greater selection of media examples which reflect the enhanced visibility of mental illness. This includes many instances of autobiographical writing, film portrayals or soap characters that portray more clearly the lived and felt experience.

The relationship between society and the media has a middle ground where these participants are seen to merge. Media providers can be seen as holding a duality of roles, in a sense sitting on both sides of the relationship by transmitting as well as receiving messages. Despite this there is a sense of separateness highlighted by McQuail's view that: 'The media constitutes a separate social institution within society, with its own rules and practices, but is subject to definition and limitation by the wider society' (McQuail 2000: 5). This is where media providers might stand outside their normal sphere of influence and set of values and beliefs and engage instead within the pressures, influences or expectations engendered by their media group. It is also a place where, for example, newspaper reporters might be swayed towards a particular style of narrative (irrespective of their own held views) because of its expected attractiveness to a group of readers.

The nature of the relationship between society and the media has to some degree changed with modern resources and new interactive technologies, in a sense bringing the two groups even closer together. Certainly, the present selection of media types offers almost unlimited choice with less direct influence being exerted by media providers upon a mass audience (McQuail 2005). It is a relationship determined by a number of factors such as lifestyle or the sub-groups that individuals belong to. The intensity or degree of interaction with various media types is worthy of exploration, particularly concerning the theme of active versus passive interaction. Media providers have a clear view in mind as to the needs or requirements of their targeted audience. We make choices as to which types of media we engage with or how we access them based upon issues such as the attractiveness of a given product or the extent to which our particular needs are met. Certainly some genres are specifically geared to a fast and impactful engagement (e.g. tabloid newspapers) among their recipients compared to others that offer a more informed and detailed perusal (e.g. broadsheet newspapers). Daytime television, for instance, serves up a diet of soaps and chat shows which are geared towards a less involved interaction. Viewers are engaged through a fast turnover of themes and sub-plots and can quite comfortably follow programmes with only partial attention. Media types such as film are different whereby messages are presented as a collective and total package requiring a more involved and responsive degree of attention from their audience. New media brings with it a fresh degree of choice, especially with the potential for a fast accessibility of a wide array of resources.

Media providers spend considerable sums of money in studying the needs of their targeted audiences and seeking further ways of enhancing audience engagement with their products. An audience's requirements are multi-faceted and might either relate to their needs to be entertained for purposes of relaxation, stimulation and distraction or to be educated for reasons such as a desire to learn, satisfying curiosity, or being reassured. Increased competition and financial considerations place further pressures upon media groups to engage consumers. This leads to the use of techniques that make messages stand out from the background, such as powerful and emotive newspaper headlines or overly dramatic scenes in television shows.

The media's relationship with mental health issues

Media organisations are made up of individuals who belong to the same sub-groups in society as discussed earlier and naturally are prone to the same array of influences. A point worth highlighting here is that media personnel will naturally include those with personal experiences of mental health problems (self, family or friends), health care providers, as well as those with little direct contact or experience. These individuals will clearly differ in their attitudes and feelings towards the mentally ill and can be found in varied groups within the broad classification which we know as *the media*. The particular mix of people within different organisations as well as the positions of power and influence held will determine the resultant relationship between the media and mental health issues.

There are various factors which have a bearing upon how mental health themes are covered and which can be looked at with regards to whose needs are primarily being addressed. This covers issues such as commercialism and mental health promotion.

Commercialism

What is clearly of great interest to various media providers is the realisation that 'madness' sells. Dramatic storylines such as Sarah's obsessional and violent infatuation with Martin Fowler in *Eastenders* or *Coronation Street*'s 'Mad Maya', the deranged solicitor, all help to keep viewers gripped and in turn enhances television ratings. Likewise, the overdramatic psychopathic killer served up through numerous metamorphoses in the 'slasher' film genre has proved exceedingly popular at the box office and encourages the production in some cases of multiple sequels (Wahl 1995). Other notable examples can be found within the tabloid press where an over-dramatisation of stories helps to create maximum impact on their readers and to sell papers. The issue of commercialism therefore means that many pressures will be placed upon media personnel to frame products in a certain way. The drive towards impactful and profit-making media products means that the feelings and sensitivities of the mentally ill are largely overlooked and that guidelines and regulatory standards are ignored. There is clearly much pressure being brought to bear from within the media industry itself from editorial staff, producers and directors to produce material that enhances the commercial appeal of the product being produced.

Health promotion

As addressed above it seems as if the predominant needs being met are those of the media providers themselves. There is scope though to use various media products as vehicles to carry health promotional material. There are a number of notable examples both factual as well as fictional that help to educate the public and challenge attitudes towards 'mental illness'. Initiatives such as the Royal College of Psychiatry's (RCP 2001) Changing Minds campaign, media mental health awards and autobiographical writing all help to raise awareness of the real issues connected with mental illness. It is assisted by media products that reach large audiences, thereby gaining heightened exposure for the issues being addressed. This might include a mental health storyline depicted in television soaps such as that of the self-harming storyline which appeared in *Hollyoaks*. While clearly providing a sense of gain for the media provider, there is also a sense of what the audience can learn about the lived experience and feelings of those involved. The approach of education and promotion is furthered by *new media* products such as the Internet, which offer many opportunities for consumer updating with fast, accessible access to information available (Christensen and Griffiths 2000).

A notable development involves the degree of liaison being developed between the media and professional/service-user groups. This incorporates degrees of involvement from production of media products and consultancy support through to the creation of guidelines or feedback to media groups. Many of these groups, as can be seen with the Royal College of Psychiatry, the British Psychological Society, Mind and Mental Health Media, all provide specific training for their members to get involved with the media. The essence of all this is the mounting of a challenge to the overwhelmingly negative depiction and stigmatising portrayal of mental health issues in the media. The concept of liaison is vital as the channels of communication used by various media providers are needed in order to achieve the highest levels of exposure possible.

Society, the media and mental health issues

Finally, we can draw all these participants together to gain a sense of the total relationship which can be regarded in terms of a connecting or a distancing type. This relates to ways in which we interact with mental health issues as a consequence of media exposure either by being drawn towards them and feeling more in tune with aspects involved or of being repelled and removed to a greater distance. The *connecting/distancing* framework will be addressed in some detail throughout this book as it plays a major part in influencing the ways in which subsequent messages are formulated.

Connectors

This in a sense forms what might be seen as the lesser evoked strand (versus its more familiar stigmatising opposite) although it can likewise have an extremely powerful resonance with its audience. It is here that we are drawn towards certain areas of understanding and experience that are normally held at some distance because of feelings of trepidation, anxiety, or simply lack of opportunity. What is clear is that, if engaged with, there are many occasions where connecting and more empathic relationships can be fostered.

Some of these examples incorporate the somewhat striking perspective of being *inside looking out*. This is where the audience member is invited to enter the inner world of thoughts and feelings of those experiencing mental health problems. It is potentially a place where much learning can take place as well as somewhere that may for some prove uncomfortable and difficult to stay with. An example of this might be found with the first-person narrative of the psychopathic killer Patrick Bateman as related in the book *American Psycho*. There are countless, wonderful opportunities to gain real degrees of insight that can be quite striking when compared with what was previously known or 'assumed' learning concerning mental health issues. Notable examples include the film *A Beautiful Mind* and the sense of extreme confusion regarding the distinction between fantasy and reality encountered by John Nash. The clever film structure ensures that we as the audience are also able to experience the visual hallucinations and are left feeling unsure as to what is real and what is not. Another example can be seen with the fragmented and disconnected thought processes conveyed in Doris Lessing's *Briefing for a Descent into Hell*. Again, it is presented through first-person prose which keeps the reader very closely engaged with the principal character and his steady reconnection with the world around him. Also, television soaps and dramas provide examples where familiar and liked characters encounter mental health problems. These examples provide the recipient with a journey towards a closer and more engaged connection with how mental health issues are experienced by those most affected.

Distancers

This category contains by far the predominant number of mental health examples. It is where the emphasis for the audience is upon entertaining, shocking or exciting and messages are handled in thoughtless and somewhat insensitive ways with little attention given to how far they might stray from what is factual. Two particularly negative types of depiction are when the 'mentally ill' are presented either as violent figures to heighten dramatic tension, or as comic eccentricities to provide us with a sense of amusement. With regard to the former strand, examples such as the packaging of news stories provide us with numerous 'factual' associations which connect mental illness with a heightened propensity for violence. This is evidenced in the style of writing using jargonistic and emotive words and narrative (Philo 1996b). This connection is further reinforced through a steady stream of examples evidenced across all media types including television dramas (Wilson *et al.* 1999) or the extremely powerful and popular films *Psycho* and *The Silence of the Lambs*.

Comedy is another much-used vehicle for incorporating mental health themes in order to heighten an audience's sense of amusement. Mental health issues provide us with the full range of characterisations from the likeable eccentric, as seen in the cinematic examples of *Harvey* and *Arsenic and Old Lace*, through to the unlikeable or offensive, in particular Jim Carrey's character in *Me, Myself and Irene*. Perhaps the key distinction with these varied examples is the degree to which we are engaged in either laughing *at* or *with* those depicted as 'mentally ill'. However, whichever way we regard this issue, these stereotypical representations serve to perpetuate the sense of difference perceived between those with mental health problems and the rest of the population.

There are also considerations whereby recipients fluctuate between the states of connecting and distancing. One of the factors influencing the public's distancing response is that of reaching a place which feels less threatening or uncertain. We might be exposed for a short space of time to a person's lived experience although then opt to remove ourselves to a more comfortable distance. For example, the reading of an autobiographical account of a person's struggling with a life of sexual abuse has the potential to evoke feelings of sympathy and horror. It connects us with uncomfortable and distressing feelings as well as a sense of helplessness where it may be easier to detach from what we are being exposed to and psychologically move away.

Why the need for this book?

The need for this book is highlighted through numerous studies that indicate the predominantly negative depiction being portrayed by the media. An overwhelming array of stigmatising imagery and negative associations can be found in media examples throughout history to the present day. This book fits within the current climate where a greater number of studies, campaigns and initiatives are being set up to challenge the negative representation and increase the positive promotion of mental health. These approaches are helping to replace some of the traditionally held, stereotypical ideas with more helpful and less alienating ones. Essentially, as addressed above, it brings us closer to the term *mental illness* in every respect, permitting us to actually gain a greater sense of what is involved. The need therefore is to appreciate how attitudes and understanding of mental health issues are shaped and fostered through exposure to varied media products. This involves examining the influences affecting both the sender (media provider) and the recipient (audience) and the nature of the resultant relationship with mental health issues, either of a connecting or distancing type.

The need to address how the media reflect and address mental health issues is clearly identified by a number of prominent studies and reports. Media representations of mental health issues would appear in the main to be increasingly portraying negative images and comment, and concerns about this have been expressed by many groups including governmental, professional and mental health service-user organisations (Health Education Authority 1999; Mind 2000; Mindout for Mental Health 2001a; Day and Page 1986). These all highlight the need for further attention and, despite some movement in the right direction, the media as a whole still requires a much greater emphasis upon positive promotion. It involves beginning to change the current picture to one which is more real, one that reflects what is really going on, such as the fact that the mentally ill are more at risk from the general public than vice versa.

The current picture does provide some heartening developments especially with regard to stigma minimisation and the media. Commissioned by the Department of Health, Mindout for Mental Health (2001a) is working closely with partners in the voluntary sector, the media, companies and youth and student organisations to combat the stigma and discrimination surrounding mental health. It includes:

- Running workshops for journalists and media professionals on portraying mental health issues in the media
- Producing a practical guide on mental health in the media for trainee journalists

This fits in with the positive mental health promotion urged by the National Service Framework (DOH 1999) standard which outlines: '[a need to] promote mental health for all . . . combat discrimination against individuals and groups with mental health problems, and promote social inclusion' (DOH 1999). A number of initiatives instigated by mental health professionals include the Royal College of Psychiatrists (2001) five years (1998–2003) anti-stigma campaign 'Changing Minds: Every Family in the Land'. One of the aims of the Changing Minds campaign is to challenge the inaccurate representation of mental illness in the media and elsewhere, based on stigmatising attitudes and stereotypes, myths, misunderstandings and discriminatory attitudes.

There is some evidence of change as highlighted by studies carried out by the Health Education Authority in 1997 (*Making Headlines: Mental Health and the National Press*) and 1999 (*Media Mentality*) which provide a useful comparison. The 1997 study found 46 per cent of all mental health press coverage being about crime, harm to others and self-harm. Also, 40 per cent of daily tabloid articles contained stigmatising words like 'nutter' and 'loony'. The later study in 1999 found a continued fuelling of stigma although offered increased optimism with more favourable coverage and a growing interest in mental health issues being highlighted. An area though of core concern is that of suicide with numerous examples being cited when suicide attempts have been influenced by media messages. It is a theme focused upon in particular throughout this book.

This book aims to stimulate questioning regarding the messages that individuals are exposed to on a daily basis. It also strives to encourage the reader to stop and challenge where their information about mental health comes from and to question the credibility of the source. What is crucial to a person's learning about mental health issues is an ability to discriminate between what is accurate and what is not and to develop a more balanced understanding of the nature and experience of mental health problems.

Content summary

Chapter 2 The role of the media

This chapter begins by outlining the scope and range of media sources and presents the core communication model used – that of Berlo (1960). This model covers the flow of communication from a source (sender) to its targeted recipient (receiver). It is related to the concepts of media provider and audience member and addresses the range of influences that play a part in shaping the eventual message which is decoded by the person accessing the message. This is related to each part of the communication process with aspects such as regulatory guidelines, media type and recipient's predisposition to certain stimuli all being covered.

Chapter 3 Stigma, labelling and social exclusion

What is *bad* about various media types is summarised and covered in this section. It begins by defining stigma and then looking at related concepts such as labelling theory, deviance and social exclusion. The effects and consequences of these types of portrayal within the media are examined in detail with thought given to some of the reasons for their perpetuation by different media providers. In part this includes a look at factors such as commercial considerations and a desire among the public to be able to engage with 'monsters' and have exposure with them in a safe way. Finally, thought is given to some of the means being employed to challenge and tackle the problem of stigma.

Chapter 4 The positive depiction of mental health issues through the media

This chapter presents a contrast to the previous one highlighting what is *good* about the media. The essence given here is that not all of the messages regarding mental health conveyed by the media are bad. Increasingly, the channels for communication within the media are also being used as vehicles for health promotion and education. It includes strategies such as the development of better liaison between media providers and mental health service-users. There is also a specific focus upon media products which enable recipients to connect and engage with the experience of mental illness as well as those that help to increase a person's understanding of the reality of mental health problems. Lastly, thought is given to some of the current initiatives being employed to maintain more progressive attitudes and approaches to the mentally ill.

Chapter 5 The press

This chapter explores the portrayal of mental health issues through the medium of news reporting. It focuses primarily upon the newsprint media with particular attention being given to the broadsheet and tabloid press as well as a look at magazine coverage. Regulation and guidelines that relate specifically to the news media are covered, such as the National Union of Journalists *Code of Conduct* (NUJ 1999) and the *Code of Practice* of the Press Complaints Commission (PCC 2005). What is interesting here is that despite some very clear guidelines concerning issues such as accuracy and discrimination, stigmatising and stereotypical reporting styles continue to proliferate. The framework of headlines, narrative and imagery is applied as a means of examining some of the broad differences between publication types.

Chapter 6 Literature

The depiction of mental health issues through the medium of literature is reflected upon here with the different publication types of autobiography, semi-autobiography and fiction being covered. It begins with a look at historical sources tracing the portrayal from ancient works by Homer and Virgil through to more contemporary writers such as Marge Piercy (*Woman on the Edge of Time*) and Iain Banks (*The Wasp Factory*). It addresses some of the core strengths offered by this particular medium including the ability to engage the reader more directly with the inner world of those experiencing mental health problems. The clear distinction between examples depicting mental illness as a destructive entity and those which portray it as a survivable condition is also addressed.

Chapter 7 Film

This chapter reviews the medium of film and the very diverse range of examples being reflected. The framework of narrative, sound and imagery is used to explore the way in which mental health themes are handled. Cinematic depictions can be regarded as falling within the broad categories which regard the mentally ill as: killer; afflicted genius; and comic eccentric. These are covered in detail including thought as to the range of emotions (e.g. fear, sympathy and amusement) evoked for the viewer by these distinctly different variations. It also focuses upon historical themes which reflect the changing ways in which mental health care and the mentally ill have been viewed over the years.

Chapter 8 Television

This chapter begins by considering the broad range of television programming through which we are exposed to mental health issues. Although broadly falling within factual and fictional categories there are numerous genres appealing to many different audience types. Standards and regulations which play a part in governing what is shown on television are reviewed along with the various influences that lead programme makers into neglecting them and including discriminatory content. Attention is given to some of the ways in which viewers' perceptions are shaped through the wide variety of positive and negative imagery they are exposed to. There is also discussion given to the extent to which programmes balance the aspects of entertainment and education, especially given the pressures to promote and protect audience viewing figures.

Chapter 9 The Internet

This chapter provides an opportunity to look at a modern and rapidly developing media source, that of the Internet. A major strength of this facility is the accessibility and ready availability of material providing advice, guidance and information. The scope is almost limitless covering a number of quality sites run by professional groups and user-carer organisations as well as a range of unregulated and poorly constructed ones. The quality varies greatly from those that are informative to those that are misleading. Some of the attempts at providing markers of quality are reviewed including examples of kitemarking and various frameworks for rating sites. Other aspects covered include the coverage of suicide, future implications for the health care relationship and the potential offered by online therapy.

Chapter 10 And . . .?

This section draws the key themes together looking at the implications and significance for those involved with different media sources as well as health care providers. It looks at ways in which further progress can be made in improving the depiction of mental health issues across all media types. Some of the core frameworks used throughout this book are revisited and considered with regards to ongoing development. These are the themes of connecting; educating and exposure. Essentially it relates to ways in which better relationships can be fostered between society and the topic *mental health*.

2 Media sources and the role of the media

Introduction

This chapter is about the flow of communication from a media source to its audience. It addresses the multiplicity of processes and influences that play a part in shaping the message which is finally received. Numerous aspects come into play regarding each stage of the communication process from the initial processing and framing of information to be sent out, the channel along which it is transmitted and its eventual reception and decoding. In a number of cases the message sent out may alter significantly to the one which is received. The reasons for this, such as the differing perspectives between sender and receiver, will be examined later on in detail.

We have on the one hand a sender or transmitter of information and on the other a recipient. The message relayed between them, in the context of this book, relates to mental health content. This subject matter can be very powerfully emotive with opinions being very clearly divided dependent upon expectations and experience. For example, a group of people might watch the film *Me Myself and Irene* yet differ wildly in how they receive it with some finding it 'entertaining' and 'hilarious' while others regard it as 'insulting' or 'totally misleading'. Of significance within this process are the reasons behind the media provider's intentions and subsequent packaging of their product as well as the audience member's personal viewpoint and interpretation of the received messages. These issues are all addressed in detail using Berlo's (1960) communication model (see Figure 2.1) as the framework for examining the flow of data from one source to another.

The core components of Berlo's (1960) communication model are:

- referent (the stimulus which begins the communication process)
- sender (the initiator of contact)
- message (information or data which is sent or expressed)
- medium (channel) (the vehicle for transmission of messages)
- receiver (recipient and interpreter of message sent)
- and feedback (response to sender).

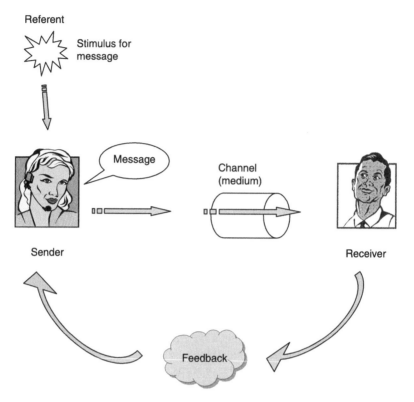

Figure 2.1 The communication process. Adapted from Berlo's communication model (1960).

Referent

The referent refers to the stimulus or purpose for any given communication process (Berlo 1960). In this case the needs of the media provider or alternatively those of the consumer can be seen as constituting the main driving force. What these needs are will clearly differ and there may be a strong feeling of conflict between these two groups. It is therefore hard to ascertain the degree to which the needs and requirements of each are being satisfied. We can also consider the pressure or influence from other parties whereby media messages are carried on behalf of external sources and organisations such as political parties, advertisers, lobbyists, businesses, social action groups and government departments (McQuail 1997). The following addresses the media provider's requirements concerning commercial and therapeutic gain as well as the consumer's need for entertainment or education.

The media provider's need

The term *media provider* here is a vastly encompassing description which includes a diverse collection of individuals. Tension may obviously exist at this stage between the different needs of those involved such as the consummatory and instrumental tension identified by Berlo (1960). For instance, a tabloid journalist might seek recognition as a credible writer (consummatory intention) by producing a clear and honest article yet is pressured by the editor who is concerned with sales (instrumental intention) to adopt a jargon-filled and moralistic style of writing.

For the *media provider* as a group entity, one of the prime factors relating to the inclusion of mental health material relates to financial considerations. The inclusion of mental health content adds an extra touch of drama that has an influence upon box office takings, television ratings, as well as newspaper and book sales. 'Madness' as a topic is both fascinating and compelling and has proved immensely attractive to many different audiences. This provides media organisations with strong incentives to include mental health content even though it may result in poor quality products. Wahl (1995) reflects this point with the example of the many 'slasher' films being made with multiple sequels, each seemingly worse than the preceding one because of the tendency of investors to repeat what has proved profitable in the past.

It is also worth noting the manner in which the referent for mental health coverage is 'located' by some media providers within their audience. Instead of openly recognising the profitability of such content, the public's need to know is cited as being the most salient aspect. Whether the need was there in the public domain in the first place or whether it was created by the media is a point of contention. For example, tabloid newspaper coverage would have an uninformed observer believing that the public have an apparently insatiable appetite to hear more about David and Victoria Beckham as well as other popular celebrities. The headlines, column inches and pictures given up to these individuals in many cases far exceed the newsworthiness of their actual exploits. It is as if the public is being offered an extremely limited menu from which to choose from as well as being led to what to access. This is reflected in other media formats such as the heavy scheduling on television of 'reality' shows which proliferate the daily schedules. High ratings are obtained for programmes which place characterless individuals in situations where little of note which is unmanufactured occurs.

There are other reasons for including mental health content such as where individuals have a vested interest in health promotion initiatives or personal therapeutic gain. There has been a steady increase over the past few years in mental health service-user groups becoming involved in a range of media projects and initiatives. The stimulus is provided through the need to promote education and engagement of the general public towards developing less stigmatising and better informed attitudes. From an educational point of view, Internet sites, booklets, fact sheets and television documentaries present just a small selection of what is available. Engagement is also achieved through creative and expressive forms such as art exhibitions, film festivals (e.g. the Royal College of Psychiatrists' Mind Odyssey) and various dramatic productions. The main stimulus here is provided by the potential change that can be brought about in the receiver. As well as gain for the receiver, there is a potential therapeutic benefit for the creator of a media product. An example can be seen in literature with the ever-increasingly popular autobiographical genre and the approach of *writing as therapy*. The act of writing here provides the author with an opportunity to work through and make sense of individual trauma thereby gaining much personally through the process of writing. There is a duality of purpose here as many autobiographical products reach wide audiences and have a high marketable value. This can be seen with Dave Pelzer's writing about his experience of being abused as a child (beginning with *A Child Called It*) and his subsequent coming to terms with it through a series of hugely popular books.

It is hard therefore to separate out exactly what the catalyst for this process is although we can see from the sender's point of view a number of incentives for the inclusion of mental health material. These incorporate gains for the sender in terms of financial incentives, opportunities for educating the public as well as therapeutic gain through the process of constructing media products.

The consumer's need

The diversity of consumers' needs can be viewed through two separate categories, those of education and entertainment.

Education

A NEED TO BE INFORMED

The importance of the media as a primary communicating agent regarding mental illness is highlighted by Sieff (2003). As consumers, our need for information about mental health issues is stimulated by factors such as personal mental health experience, curiosity about a compelling and fascinating topic, or a need for reassurance. Personal experience of mental health problems will certainly create a desire to seek out information concerning support groups, available treatments and the nature of specific conditions. If we take for instance the example of somebody who has recently been diagnosed with depression a core resource accessed might be the Internet. It is a medium that is proving ever more attractive to mental health service-users because of the ready accessibility and availability of information (Scrivener 2002). Alternatively, they might seek out some of the many self-help books or autobiographical accounts available such as Andrew Solomon's (2002) informative and insightful *The Noonday Demon – an Anatomy of Depression* which was voted Mind's book of the year in 2002. This publication combines an autobiographical account of the experience of depression along with a critical review of the available evidence, concerning causal factors and treatment approaches. The main issue however relates to the ability that individuals have in selecting from the wide range of resources available, discriminating between what is informative and helpful and what is misleading and potentially harmful.

As well as accessing information for health reasons it is worth also considering the desire of many people to satisfy their own interest or curiosity in what is potentially a compelling and fascinating yet much misunderstood topic. Soap storylines, documentaries, magazine articles, novels and newspaper reports form just a small part of the many different products carrying a mental health theme that are available. In the main they are very popular and marketable, in many cases engaging their audience more for entertainment than for purposes of education.

A NEED FOR REASSURANCE

One of the strands relating to informational needs is governed by feelings of anxiety and discomfort about the mentally ill. It is a need created in part by the media themselves through sensational, explicit and emotive reporting that all serve to unsettle their audience. For example, the saturation coverage of a high-profile crime involving a perpetrator with mental health problems usually evokes a desire for reassurance and understanding. In particular, people seek to find out how such horrific acts might have been prevented. Fears abound centring on aspects such as whether any tell-tale signs were in evidence as to an individual's potential for violence. The apparent demand for information is met in abundance by the media and in some cases involves extraneous fine detail. It seems there is little which is not covered and one often wonders about the degree of insensitivity being shown especially to the families of those concerned. The message being conveyed is that we as a public need to know and want to know all of these intricate details. Because people with mental health problems often do not display any noticeable traits, unlike the traits or characteristics which are often grossly exaggerated within much of the fictional media, it seems that our need for reassurance is enhanced. As the general public are unable to adequately spot who poses a risk to their community, the focus becomes all encompassing. Therefore all those who have the label 'mental illness' applied to them become included within the mass of individuals from whom a general sense of threat is felt.

Entertainment

This covers different elements and may be seen to include a desire for both humorous as well as frightening imagery.

A NEED TO LAUGH

Laughter is important for many reasons including stimulation, stress relief and relaxation. From a mental health point of view the outcast or the fool has historically provided a focus for derision or merriment and can be seen within countless comical depictions. The characterisation ranges from the harmless eccentric (James Stewart's alcoholic character in the film *Harvey*) through to the grossly misrepresented and shameless depictions (Jim Carrey's Hank/Charlie in *Me, Myself and Irene*). We are enticed towards either laughing *with* the character or perhaps in a number of instances laughing *at* them. It is the latter portrayal which is more harmful, undermining much of the work done to combat stigmatising and stereotypical portrayals. Some examples are grossly insensitive and fail to recognise the real seriousness of the subject matter being depicted. A prime example of this is the *Viz* adult cartoon strip character Suicidal Sid, who cheerfully engages in a number of seemingly comic ways to try and kill himself. Unfortunately, the comic clown proves very popular to consumers and appears regularly in derisive imagery and jargonistic language. It shows an overall lack of responsibility by media providers that they are prepared to offer products which are beneficial to them but at the expense of those being ridiculed. Certainly one could argue that many instances contain examples that are simply harmless fun, although they all play a part in developing a global picture that entails those with mental health problems not being taken seriously.

A NEED TO BE SCARED

This need provides the impetus for the increasingly popular horror genre. Films and books of every conceivable quality are produced in order to meet an almost insatiable demand. The principal attraction is the opportunity to experience strong emotions such as terror in a secure and contained environment. We are simultaneously brought into close contact with fearful stimuli as well as retaining a comfortably safe distance. Mental illness adds an extra level of intensity to the fearful scenes being depicted and heightens the experience felt. Mad killers are far more frightening because of their depiction as frenzied or unpredictable. Their ranks include cannibal killers (*The Silence of the Lambs* and *The Texas Chain Saw Massacre*), apparently indestructible killers (*Halloween*), phantom-like killers (*Nightmare on Elm Street* and Freddie Krueger). Perhaps the most frightening are those who are portrayed as apparently normal until their madness becomes apparent. There are two classic Hitchcock examples here involving Norman Bates as the nervy motel owner in *Psycho* and Barry Foster as the affable and confident character in *Frenzy*. A core aspect with these portrayals is the ability the recipient has in putting the book down, leaving the cinema or turning the television off. It is a means of experiencing cathartically strong emotions which we would be unable to do otherwise. The highly popular nature of this form of enter-tainment means that many new examples are being created.

Sender

The types of message being packaged and transmitted by media groups are subject to a variety of factors and influences. First, the particular character-istics of a given media provider and the available channel of communication will play a significant part in shaping the message to be sent out. Of particu-lar relevance is the influence exerted by those who hold a controlling influence in a given media type. This is further affected by the degree of control and structuring exerted through regulation and censorship of media products. This may be set up through internal procedures whereby a media provider has a self-regulatory approach or as a response to pressure from outside agencies such as governmental legislation. There are also various types of guidance provided for those working within media organisations from a range of men-tal health groups (professional and service-user) aimed at achieving a better portrayal of mental health issues.

Ownership

One of the most significant factors influencing the media relates to the con-cept of ownership. Whether media organisations are set up as profit making or non-profit making ventures or are private or public concerns, the concept of ownership has a strong bearing upon media content (Devereux 2003). If we consider the global picture, mainstream media ownership progressively rests in fewer hands as a consequence of mergers, takeovers, technological change and privatization. This results in a concentration of ownership with a handful of national and multinational corporations dominating the mass communications industry (Bagdikian 1997). At the same time conglomer-ation has been taking place, with media companies becoming part of larger corporations which in turn grow bigger. A major influencing factor is that in concentrated media ownership the search for profit is seen as key arbiter of what is produced (O'Sullivan, Dutton and Rayner 1994). Croteau and Hoynes (2000) reflect upon the impact of conglomeration in that previously some news media had been sheltered from the full pressure of profit making. This view is supported by Squires (1993), who indicates that corporate take-overs of print media place an emphasis upon entertaining and attracting consumers rather that informing them. All of this has major implications with regard to the reporting of mental health issues as sensitivity and realism are not as appealing from a sales perspective as are the usual stereotypical 'fodder' served up by large sections of the media.

The small number of controlling interests with regard to the mass media results in audiences becoming conditioned to accept a somewhat limited view of the world (McQuail 2005). This picture is changing with the increased choice currently being offered by the rise and development of new media products and services (cable and satellite, fibre optic technology and computers) and has resulted in a move away from mass broadcast audiences towards smaller, more specialised niche populations. It is a process described by Croteau and Hoynes (2000) as 'narrowcasting' and provides a contrast to the conglomeration of media providers. The implications here are that a greater degree of choice can be offered to consumers concerning the type of media products available. The greater flexibility and choice of media services and products also means that the concept of ownership is increased to include a greater number of individuals and organisations with a vested interest in mental health issues. For example, a brief search for mental health related material on the Internet indicates a wide array of information that has been posted by professional organisations, service-user groups and individuals with an experience of mental health problems.

Censorship

Each media source explored within this book will be examined with a focus upon the constraints or structures that play a fundamental part in shaping the message to be sent out. The pressure brought to bear upon media providers comes from many different sources with varying degrees of authority. We can first look at the process of internal regulation, whereby a degree of control is exerted by the media organisation itself or those working within it, i.e. writers, producers or editors. Second, we can refer to the range of external regulations that are imposed by various authoritative bodies and which include governmental legislation.

One form of regulation is provided through censorship, whereby products are gauged regarding their suitability for public consumption. The term *censorship* has different connotations and can be welcomed on the one hand as a necessary safeguard protecting vulnerable groups in society (i.e. children), or alternatively might be seen as an oppressive and controlling power curtailing freedom of speech. Censorship is applied with the rationale and explanation that it is the public's interest that is being served. Many examples of censorship can be found across different media formats with examples such as the books *Lady Chatterley's Lover* and *Lolita* or the films *Crash* and *The Man with the Golden Arm*. In many instances what is deemed acceptable or unacceptable differs according to the perspective with which a product is viewed. First, we might consider a historical perspective as what is deemed unsuitable in one era may be perfectly acceptable at a later date. A clear example of this is the 1954 Marlon Brando film *The Wild One* which was not screened in Britain until 1968 for the damaging effect it was felt it might have upon young people watching it. Interestingly, by today's standards the mean and moody posturing of Brando's motorcycle gang appears more camp and comedic. Another important aspect is the issue of cultural acceptability as different groups of people hold contrasting views over, for example, religious or moral grounds. This has been seen in the hostile reception by certain groups to some media products, such as the fatwa ordered over Salman Rushdie's *Satanic Verses* or the viewing of Monty Python's *A Life of Brian* which was regarded as blasphemous and offensive.

A major factor is of course the question as to exactly whose interests are being served through censorship. From a political point of view, curtailing free speech might be regarded as a necessary means of controlling a populace. This can be seen in a number of examples such as during China's Cultural Revolution or in the eastern bloc communist regimes where censorship was applied as a means of silencing particular expressions and controlling people's thoughts and speech. In some cases it was severely applied, in its most drastic forms resulting in imprisonment, exile or even execution. The effects upon those censored are well documented in a number of sources including Jung Chang's powerful autobiographical novel *Wild Swans*, which documents the harsh and restrictive climate that existed within Mao's China.

One might argue that a counter-productive outcome from censorship is that in a number of instances it has the opposite desired effect. It can draw attention to and effectively promote the product it is trying to restrict. In other words, censorship instils a sense of power and attractiveness in products that may not have been there in the first place. The perhaps short-sighted approach of banning radio air time to the Sex Pistols' *God Save the Queen* or Frankie goes to Hollywood's *Relax* made both of these records instant hits. Another example can be seen in the huge sales of D.H. Lawrence's novel *Lady Chatterley's Lover* that immediately followed its initial banned publication.

Clearly censorship has different applications pertinent to the place and media type. In England for example, there is no direct censorship of the written word although any publication can be challenged in the courts 'after the event'. Published work could be challenged for instance by legislative acts relating to issues of obscenity, blasphemy or racial hatred. Therefore in labelling a book as obscene one would need to show that it tended to 'deprave' or 'corrupt' the reader. This clearly though relates to the targeted audience as what might not be an obscene publication for an adult might easily be held to be obscene and tasteless if made available to children. As far as mental health issues go, it is far less clear and it seems that there is no clear legislation protecting this group. Using the previous example, what is deemed to be stigmatising and harmful by those experiencing mental health problems might differ considerably from the views or perceptions of the general public. The difficulty in changing this picture lies in the attractiveness and appeal that the topic of *madness* has for media providers and consumers alike. Products that are grossly offensive or harmful provide greater opportunities for seeking redress from their instigators, although the large numbers that are 'merely' insensitive or misleading are harder to tackle.

Media regulations and guidelines

Depending upon the media format type, there are different sets of guidelines and regulatory standards that govern the type of message to be sent out. Television, for example is heavily regulated with particular advice regarding mental health content provided initially by the Broadcasting Standards Commission *Codes of Guidance* (1998) and the Independent Television Commission *Programme Code* (2002), but now assumed by Ofcom. With regard to 'the Press', the *Code of Practice* of the Press Complaints Commission (UK) (2005) and the National Union of Journalists (1999) *Code of Conduct* highlight the need for journalists to ensure accuracy and fairness in their writing and to avoid discrimination. The cinematic world is influenced by bodies such as the British Board of Film Classification (BBFC) and the Motion Picture Association of America (MPAA) that have a role in classifying films regarding their suitability to various audience groups. Even largely unregulated 'new media' formats such as the Internet are beginning to create indicators of quality (such as the Hon Code), which include approved evidence based sites. Ofcom, the regulator for the UK communication industries has been given responsibility for 'maintaining content standards in the electronic media'. Guidance even extends to the world of advertising where the Advertising Standards Authority (ASA) administers the various Codes of Advertising across a range of broadcast and non-broadcast media. The Disability Discrimination Act (1995), although including the term *mental impairment*, does not feature strongly with regard to mental health issues as there is little evidence of it being applied in instances other than those concerning physical impairment.

One mental health theme in particular, around which a considerable range of guidelines have been produced, is that of suicide. The Department of Health (2002) has produced a consultation document *National Suicide Prevention Strategy for England*, which sets out a number of goals to improve the reporting of suicidal behaviour in the media. This builds upon evidence that the reporting of suicide can increase the rate especially among those already at risk (DOH 2002). It is stated that: 'By limiting some aspects of the reporting of suicide and by portraying it in ways which may discourage imitation, the media can make an important contribution to suicide prevention.' (DOH 2002:19).

Other bodies such as the Samaritans (1997) set out a structure for guidance on suicide coverage in the media which includes:

- Avoid sensationalism and remove positive messages about suicide
- Avoid reference to suicide
- Increase the prominence given to responsible reports on suicide prevention
- Include facts about suicide
- Influence the training of journalists to ensure that they report on mental illness and suicidal behaviour in an informed and sensitive manner

- Establish a method of ensuring that such training is repeated in a rolling programme

Perhaps one of the most striking features is that despite each media provider having its own set of guidelines that regulate against the employment of discriminating or stigmatising imagery, there seem to be only small movements being made to reduce the steady stream of negative and stigmatising depictions. It seems that the incentives for producing ever-more impactful and commercially enticing products in many instances prove stronger than those of respecting and adhering to available regulatory guidelines.

Training and media involvement

A notable development over recent years has been the gradual increase in direct involvement that health care professionals and mental health service-user groups have fostered with various media providers. This particularly relates to the broadcast and print media and encompasses a variety of roles such as the offering of comment and consultancy services or through direct involvement with production. As a consequence, many professional and service-user groups now offer training and advice to their members who are wishing to become more proactively engaged with the media. It has been furthered through initiatives such as the Department of Health's (2001) Mindout for Mental Health's (2001a) Mindshift campaign and the Royal College of Psychiatrists' (2001) Changing Minds campaign that have targeted the need to reduce stigmatising media coverage of mental health issues and include recommendations for the development of greater collaboration between mental health groups and media providers. The importance of this type of liaison cannot be overestimated as it means that media personnel are provided with informed guidance and are called upon to question what they are producing. One notable example is the collaborative *Guide for Journalists and Broadcasters Reporting on Schizophrenia* produced, among other parties, by the Royal College of Psychiatrists and the National Union of Journalists.

Berlo

Berlo (1960) identifies 4 factors within the source which play a part in increasing the fidelity of the communication process: Communication skills, attitudes, knowledge level, and position within a socio-cultural system.

Communication skills

The type of communication utilised within the media is influential here and may take many forms including those of a written, narrative, visual or sound base. The expressiveness and complexity of a message will clearly be increased through the use of multiple forms. Also, the recipient's favoured mode of address needs to be borne in mind.

Attitudes

The attitudes of the sender towards self, subject matter and the receiver all play a significant part here. One of the main strands would be the relationship that media personnel have with the issue of mental illness. For example, the message sent out from someone with personal experience of mental health problems may be shaped much more sensitively than from somebody with little or no awareness. Media personnel clearly have some expectations as to what the perceived consumer's needs are and will gear presentations towards specific recipient groups. An example of this can be seen in the press and the type of language used as well as the way in which news stories are constructed and formatted.

Knowledge level

Berlo states that:

> One cannot communicate with maximum effectiveness content material that one does not understand. On the other hand if the source knows too much, if he is overspecialized, he might err in that his particular communication skills are employed in so technical a manner that his receiver cannot understand him.
>
> (Berlo 1960: 48)

This statement raises a number of issues which can be addressed with regard to the handling of information by the media. The first part of this statement certainly does not deter a lot of misleading and erroneous presentation that can be found within numerous media products, much of which would seem to suggest that the originator of the message does not indeed know much about the subject they are portraying. It may be that media providers in some instances are acting in good faith with the information they are presenting, although they are unable to recognise that their sources of knowledge are flawed. As Wahl (1995) points out, misconceptions that abound in the general public are shared by those involved with the media. The second strand, that of over-specialism, may be true of some examples, such as Internet sites or some health promotional material, although the question here would relate to appropriateness of different information types to their intended audience.

Position within a socio-cultural system

This category addresses all the influences upon one's perception of the world around us. The way we structure and interpret mental health issues may be borne out of personal experience or attitudinal aspects and expectations of the various groups we belong to. This includes the ways in which group pressure can play a part in the modification and distortion of judgement (Asch 1961).

Message

Message framing

One of the core features of the communicating process involves the particular way in which a message has been shaped or presented. Framing can be defined as the means by which media information is organised, presented and subsequently interpreted (Sieff 2003). This can be explored through frameworks, such as Hall's (1974a) encoding/decoding model, that address the codes and conventions employed by media professionals in the construction of messages and their subsequent decoding by audience members. These features are also outlined by Berlo (1960) who highlights the factors of:

- Message code – a group of symbols structured in a way that is meaningful to another person i.e. language, music, painting, dance
- Message content – the material in the message which provides structure
- Message treatment – the decisions which the communication source makes in selecting and arranging both codes and content. It includes what is deemed interesting to the receiver

Clearly, frequently negative frames contribute towards the public's unfavourable attitudes to issues of mental health. This may be out of context with actual reality, as outlined by Philo:

> The media are highlighting a tiny minority of cases relative to the very large number of people with mental health problems, and that in doing so media accounts are distorting public perceptions of the whole area of mental health.
>
> (Philo 1996b: xii)

This statement is disturbing in that the core message being carried by the media as a whole is incorrect and misleading. The educative and evidence based information is submerged within a larger mass which means that in many cases they will be missed or, as with Broadbent's (1958) filter theory, the weight of what is transmitted is diluted by the plethora of competing messages.

The means of communication will obviously vary according to the media type selected although broadly can be seen as comprising those of imagery, narrative and sound.

Imagery

Mental health imagery has a powerful resonance with those accessing it and often evokes strong emotions. The imagery is frequently negative with the mentally ill being portrayed as being bizarrely different or violent and dangerous. This reflects Wahl's (1995) notion of those with mental health problems being segregated and treated as 'a breed apart'. The continued need for this type of representation is perhaps reinforced because of the psychologically self-protective function it serves. In a sense this means that individuals can discriminate more simply between the mentally ill and the mentally well and therefore take steps towards what is felt to be a safe distance.

When considering the nature of images it is important to note the various ways in which they are encountered or created through both pictures and words. The essence perhaps is of audience perception as in some cases the recipient is guided towards very specific interpretations and in others might be confused by ambiguous messages and left to form much of their own understanding. Visual imagery is powerfully depicted within the media of film and television and can present viewers with pictures of what is happening within a character's internal world or what is external and observable by others. An example of the former can be seen in Polanski's *Repulsion* where the cracks appearing in the walls form symbolic representations of the principal character's fragmenting mental health state. The more commonly portrayed imagery, though, seems to be located in the second element, that of external impressions and characterisations. The predominant presentation here is of individuals who look different, such as David Helfgott's dishevelled looking character in the film *Shine* or the scary intensity of Anthony Hopkins as Hannibal Lecter.

Mental health imagery is impactful and compelling and can serve to engage the receiver in a very powerful way. These images are often negative and portray the mentally ill through a number of stereotypes such as appearing violent, socially inadequate or eccentric (Wilson *et al.* 1999). Children's media in particular abounds with stereotypical caricatures, either that of the evil madman or the drooling idiot (Wahl 2003a; Wilson *et al.* 2000). In many cases these images permeate our thinking and feelings about those we regard as mentally ill, leaving us with associations that in some instances bear little resemblance to what the reality actually is. The audience are provided with positive imagery as well although the violent and scary images are often the more potent with images of Norman Bates or Hannibal Lecter superseding other, softer ones such as Judy Dench's emotive role in the film *Iris*.

Imagery is also used to portray factors other than characterisation and includes background features such as the settings within which care is delivered. A wide contrast is presented here from the stark and sterile environment in *One Flew over the Cuckoo's Nest* and *Girl Interrupted* to the cluttered yet comfortable psychotherapists' offices in *Ordinary People* or *Good Will Hunting*. In most of these cases the environment within which scenes take place act as a secondary means of communication conveying to the audience member a feeling of mood which resembles the style of care being offered – either impersonal and severe or warm and secure. The particular choice of setting is not always apparent although we might suppose that suspenseful or dramatic engagement play a part. The film *Gothika*, for example, features a high-security mental health institution which is on reflection rather unnecessary as well as misleading. The high level of security conveys to the viewer a feeling of potential danger from those imprisoned and serves to perpetuate the age-old association between mental illness and violence potential.

Imagery is also created through the written word whereby the reader creates their own pictures from the text in front of them. In a number of cases the reader is led towards formulating their impressions through direct cues provided by the author. For example, in the book *Harry Potter and the Goblet of Fire* the madness of Mr Crouch is described to the reader through drawing attention to his dishevelled appearance and odd behaviour – 'He looked utterly mad. His eyes were rolling and bulging, and a trickle of spittle was sliding down his chin.' The image portrayed is not a positive one and connects the reader very quickly to many classic stereotypes regarding the mentally ill. The written word also creates symbolic imagery that is representative of other related aspects. Kafka's *Metamorphosis* for instance powerfully conveys the reaction of others towards disease or human suffering through the symbolic of portrayal of Gregor Samsa's plight at finding himself transformed overnight into a beetle.

Narrative

A core distinction with regard to narrative style relates to whether or not those with mental health problems are referred to by an external narrator or through first-person accounts. The former applies to much of what readers might get from newspapers or literature. The printed word can be very evocative and can build up a damning picture of individuals through a few select words such as 'psycho', 'mental' or 'schizo'. The type of words chosen may be misleading, inaccurate and damaging yet at the same time favoured by a media provider because of their ability to achieve dramatic impact. Take for instance the headlines 'Freed Cannibal Killer Ate Brain of One of his Victims' (*Daily Mirror* online version), '*Silence of the Lambs* Maniac Freed to Kill' (*Today*) and 'A Psychotic on the Loose in Suffolk' (*Guardian*). These use words in very emotive and disparaging ways that are morbidly appealing to their potential readers. It conjures up, though, very unfavourable stereotypes maintaining a range of negative associations such as that of mental illness and the potential for violence. The continued use of stereotypes is explained by Salter (2003) in that people prefer certainties and that stereotypes reduce the uncertainty accompanying new and novel stimuli.

Madness as a topic is commercially attractive and appealing to readers and the medium of literature includes numerous books which include mental health themes as a means of engagement. The predominant presentation is through third-person narratives that generally feature those with mental health problems for their interest or entertainment value. In a number of instances their inclusion represents an external threat and thereby aids the building of tension especially when we are concerned about the safety of central characters. The lurking, psychopathic presence somewhere outside helps to build the suspense to an almost unbearable tension as in books such as Patricia Cornwell's *Body of Evidence* or Ian McEwan's *Enduring Love.*

Alternatively, there is a growing body of journalistic writing and auto-biographical literature in which the author takes us beyond the surface into the thoughts and feelings of those experiencing mental health problems. In these instances words lead us on a guided tour through someone else's inner world and provide the reader with a glimpse of that person's thoughts, feelings and beliefs. It is a type of presentation that is seen frequently within magazines with articles such as 'My Drugs Hell' or 'Surviving Depression'. It has also over recent years become extraordinarily popular within the genre of autobiographical writing and often features strongly within best-selling book lists. They are written mainly from a position of survival with authors having 'come through' sometimes appalling experiences, yet they provide feelings of optimism and hope for the future. David Pelzer for example has written four extremely successful books about his experience of child abuse and the way in which he has been able to foster a healthy relationship with his own son. First-person narratives are also employed within fiction as a means of connecting the reader more closely with the inner world of characters who are experiencing mental health problems. It is a journey that is not always comfortable and can be extremely unsettling as with narratives that keep the reader engaged for an entire book within disordered (*Briefing for a Descent into Hell*) or psychopathic (*American Psycho*) worlds.

Sound

The previous two parts are concerned with the ways in which we engage with the media and interpret messages through what we see. A further powerful strand of communication can be seen in terms of what we hear, experience through music, exclamations and the spoken word. First, we can look at the use of music as a means of generating feelings among the receiver, be it peacefulness and tranquillity or a sense of imminent danger. When connected with a visual medium such as film or television, sound and music act as a vital mode of communication, informing the receiver for instance when a powerful moment is occurring and guiding them towards a particular emotional response (Turner 1999). It also has a function of amplifying the mood or atmosphere connected with a particular scene as can be seen in Hitchcock's shower scene in the film *Psycho* where the sense of danger and suspense are powerfully evoked through the unnerving and shrieking violin strings

(Carroll 1996). The type of music played in some cases provides cues to the receiver as to the underlying psychological states of characters (Prendergast 1992). Bobker (1969) provides a clear example of this in the film *Through a Glass Darkly* where the fragmentation between the music and the film scenes not quite fitting together reveal something of the daughter's schizophrenic world.

The advent of film, radio and television has brought new channels for carrying the spoken voice. It was previously left to the domain of dramatic stage productions to entertain their audience with spoken narrative regarding mental illness. There is a rich historical base here including a number of plays by Shakespeare (e.g. *King Lear* or *Macbeth*) and we can look even further back in time to the Greek tragedies such as the Euripidean dramas of *The Bacchae* and *Heracles*. The spoken word carries expressiveness that is not present in the written word with tone, inflexion, volume and pitch all being employed to convey specific meanings. There are many examples to be found in the media although unfortunately they seem predominantly to feature disparaging and stereotypical representations. For example, the viewer might be alerted towards a character's fragmented or distorted mental health state through their maniacal laughter, sudden exclamations or delusional speech. It is a much-employed stereotype often used within the genre of comedy such as with Inspector Clousseau's long-suffering boss in the Pink Panther films, clearly informing the viewers that he is having a breakdown. There are normally sharp distinctions made between the language of wellness and the language of illness. As with Wahl's (1995) concept of the mentally ill being featured as *a breed apart*, they not only look different but they also sound different. The film *Me, Myself and Irene* for instance highlights this aspect with the definite changes in vocal presentation from the well state (sensitive and quiet) to the ill state (loud and abusive). Stigmatising messages are also given through the words used by others in connection with mentally ill characters, often with demeaning and rejecting words being used. It is indeed very common to come across words such as 'fruit cake', 'nutter', 'schizo' and 'loony'. These types of portrayal perhaps stand out more forcibly from the number of examples that demonstrate a more favourable and accepting approach towards the mentally ill and fit the general stereotype and expectations of many of their audience.

Medium (channel)

Channel types

The channel of communication relates to the mode by which messages are carried between sender and receiver. Obviously attention is given to the qualities or restrictions connected with each channel type when determining how a message is to be constructed. Media channels almost exclusively cater for the senses of sight and sound, collectively covering a broad expanse of types of sensation. The visual media is experienced as pictures and words whereas sound media is conveyed predominantly through the forms of music and speech. Both cover a broad expanse of media types and are employed either as single modes of communication or are integrated to combine various stimuli more powerfully together into a unified message. The manner in which these aspects are conveyed to their audience is to a large degree determined by the type of channel they are carried by.

As media services and products continue to change so does the make up of their audience. The expanding range of media types is resulting in an audience's attention being dispersed over a number of different products and the concept of 'mass' audience is becoming more of a fragmented entity (McQuail 1997). People will belong to several different potential audiences at the same time influenced by the characteristics and attractiveness of a particular media channel. Of particular significance is the accessibility and suitability of a given channel type as it fits in with a person's daily routine. For example, one might choose to listen to the radio while driving to work or watch the television at the same time as carrying out household chores. An understanding of their audience's needs and mode of engagement is used directly by some media providers to shape and develop the product being carried. For example, the narrative form of soap operas has been linked to some of the typical features of a housewife's daily routine (fragmented and distracted) that prevent continuous attention (Geraghty 1991). Media providers therefore have in mind their audience's preference to a channel type as well as their mode of engagement with it.

The choice or selection of channel types and specific products is governed by a number of factors including those of availability, accessibility, cost implications and personal preferences. Channel sources are selected in part for what they offer over other types. For example, the Internet might be chosen instead of newspapers and books as a source of information because of the immediate access to an almost unlimited array of sites. One of the prime considerations reflects Berlo's (1960) view that communication modes are approached with a 'what's in it for me' attitude. It can also be seen in the work of Palmgreen and Rayburn (1985) that highlighted the significance of audience gratification for continued use of a particular media type. McQuail *et al.* (1972) identified a number of media–person interactions with regard to television and radio that highlight the reasons for engaging with this medium and include factors such as relaxation, diversions and companionship. There are certainly a number of aspects here that help to explain the addition of mental health content for its capacity for drama and impactful engagement, or simply as a means of drawing audience members in. This reinforces Biocca's (1988) focus upon affective arousal in that the more an audience member is 'caught up' or 'engrossed' the more they are likely to retain their engagement with a selected media type.

Media channels are also carefully chosen by those wishing to have their products carried. For instance, organisations concerned with health

promotion will have a number of factors to consider concerning which channels offer the greatest exposure. This of course is partly determined by the
financial constraints connected with each type. The expansion of new media
services and the enhanced capacity to convey a greater number of products
more cheaply is good news for mental health organisations. Traditionally, the
electronic media had proved fairly prohibitive in terms of cost although has
now opened up considerably through the financially accessible media such as
the Internet and community television channels (offered through digital and
cable television packages). The problem still exists that these more productive
and positive messages are still swamped by the plethora of stigmatising and
derogatory portrayals carried by the same channel types.

Receiver

Making sense of the media

An important framework for considering the communication between a
media provider and receiver is Hall's (1974b) encoding/decoding model. In
order to understand how a media message works or doesn't, there is a need to
explore the codes and conventions employed by media professionals in the
construction of a message and the subsequent decoding by audience members.
Hall (1974b) focuses upon four main codes:

- Dominant/hegemonic code
  The interpretation or decoding of messages by audience members in
  accordance with intended or preferred meaning.

- Professional code
  Conventions that media professionals use to encode meaning within
  media messages incorporating production techniques used to tell a story
  in a particular way.

- Negotiated code
  An audience member might accept the broad thrust of a specific media
  message yet either adapt or reject elements of the overall message
  because it does not fit with their own immediate experience of the world.

- Oppositional code
  The capacity of audience members to reject outright the preferred or
  intended meaning of a media message.

The essence of Hall's (1974b) encoding/decoding model is that a message is
constructed by a sender prior to its transmission. It is subsequently decon-
structed by the receiver although may be decoded by individual audience
members in very different ways. This is supported by Anderson (2003) who
states that some audiences will read the sender's intended meaning while
others will establish a new meaning of their own. Goffman's (1974) frame

analysis looks at the individualised nature of organising experience and the view that what one person has of what is going on is quite different from that of another. The meaning derived from media content is very dependent upon the perceptions, experiences and social location of audience members (Philo *et al.* 1994; Jensen 1988). It means in a number of cases the message encoded by the receiver is not the same as that sent out and explains to some degree the overwhelming evidence for poor or faulty understanding of news (Gunter 1987).

These aspects are reflected very aptly by White's (1990) detailing of five different people's rereading of the novel *Great Expectations*, five years after first reading it.

Reader 1: 'I loved it then, it seemed so lifelike; but now that I've studied literature I see it as a myth about bourgeois guilt about money.'

Reader 2: 'I didn't like it then, but I've seen the film since, and that made me more interested because I could visualise the scenes.'

Reader 3: 'I once found it really funny, full of macabre jokes – now it seems a complete tragedy.'

Reader 4: 'I can see more in it now – Miss Havisham is just like my aunty.'

Reader 5: 'I hated it then and I hate it now, no difference.'

White summed this up with the statement: 'On each occasion of reading, a person is a different reader bringing to the work a new set of "meanings" which he/she wants to find.' (White 1990: 250). He concludes that instead of looking for a plurality of meaning in texts we can instead look for the plurality that exists in each individual reader. Each reader therefore plays a significant part in creating the 'meaning' which they find in any given media product. This is also supported by Umberto Eco who states that: 'Every reception of a work of art is both an interpretation and a performance of it, because in every reception the work takes on a fresh perspective for itself' (Eco 1989: 4).

Another core issue for the recipient relates to their perception of a set of messages and their understanding of the context within which messages are framed. One issue relates to a person's expectations as these will clearly influence what is noticed or selected from the huge plethora of stimuli exposed to. This may entail a fair degree of wastage as most communication receives only a small fraction of its potential attention and impact (Clausse 1968). The overwhelming range of media messages sent out presents the receiver with an unmanageable supply of stimuli with which to deal. This is illustrated by Broadbent's (1958) filter theory in that what is retained by the recipient measures only a small fraction of all that is accessed. This fact clearly leads those involved in media production towards creating products that stand out from the background and gain maximum impact from their targeted audience. Mental health themes in particular can be seen as an ideal choice for inclusion because of their potential for dramatic, engaging and impactful presentations. This reflects the concept of *figure and ground* in that different interpretations can be derived from the same set of stimuli (King and Wertheimer 2005). This depends largely upon what is placed into the foreground and what is therefore relegated to the background. The illustration in Figure 2.2 may be seen either as two black silhouetted faces or a white goblet in the centre while the image in Figure 2.3 can be perceived in two very different ways, seeing either an old or young woman. Of significance here is the receiver's perspective as, for example, the impression gained of media coverage by those with first-hand experience is likely to be different from those with little or no experience.

It is also worth acknowledging the media effects model, an approach that has been used to measure the impact and influence that media products have upon those exposed to them. One of the most prominent studies is that of Bandura (1986) who illustrated the concept of social learning and how a group of children exposed to violent images developed imitative behaviour. The effects model is one that has been criticised by a number of media analysts because of its overly restrictive and linear focus which, it is felt, does not address all of the potential influencing factors (Rogers 1986). We might consider facts such as the amount of distracting 'noise' that is sent out alongside main messages or the fact that messages are open to checking through other contacts (McQuail 2005). Violent or negative images may also be responded to in alternative ways, for example being perceived as cathartic (Wolfenstein and Leites 1970; Feshbach and Singer 1971).

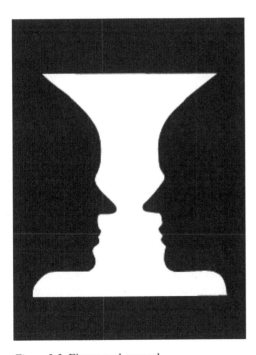

Figure 2.2 Figure and ground.

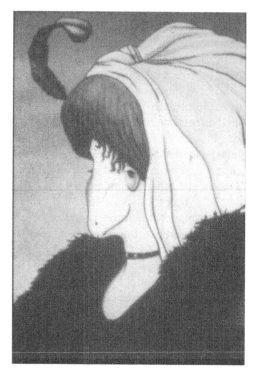

Figure 2.3 Old woman/young woman.

Feedback

Approval

This is the rounding off part to the communication cycle and one that helps to shape the ways in which messages are subsequently framed by media providers. Feedback may be received directly in the form of complaints or commendations, or indirectly through means such as box office receipts and sales figures. Perhaps the most significant factor regarding the continuation of a particular media type relates to its commercial appeal. There may in a number of instances be some discrepancy between the types of feedback received with negative comments being received alongside a product's popular receipt by large numbers of people. For example, the tabloid news press is widely regarded as having the most detrimental and stigmatising coverage of mental health issues (Mind 2000) yet at the same time receives a large percentage of the newsprint sales circulation outselling the broadsheets by far. Approval through sales in many cases appears to override the regulatory guidance and negative feedback that may be received as media types continue to produce poor representations of mental illness.

The commercial aspects are perhaps the most striking and media providers obviously have a keen eye on potential sales, ratings and box office takings. These factors first represent the continued survival of a product type but also influence aspects such as continued marketability and potential advertising revenue. High ratings and product uptake has a direct impact upon the way in which media products are constructed. The television ratings war, for example, has led to ever more dramatic storylines being developed within the popular soaps, of which mental health themes have proven very popular i.e. 'Mad Maya' in *Coronation Street*. The commercial appeal has also resulted in numerous sequels being made within the 'Psycho-killer' genre such as with the films *Nightmare on Elm Street* and *Friday the 13th*, finally bringing their murderous perpetrators together in the 2003 film *Freddy vs Jason*.

Approval is also granted for a product's content and the positive depiction of mental health issues. The annual Mental Health Media awards and the Mind Awards for the best coverage of mental health themes is one example. These highlight and showcase examples where mental health is being positively promoted. Direct feedback has been enabled through the close liaison links that have been developed by a number of media groups and mental health organisations.

Disapproval

Most media organisations provide mechanisms for complaints about their products which can be sent directly to the media body concerned or through its own specific regulatory body. For example, if concerned about items presented by the broadcast media (radio and television), individuals might contact the station or Ofcom (the office of communications). Other media with their own regulatory body include newsprint (Press Complaints Commission), the Internet (Internet Watch Foundation) and non-broadcast adverts (Advertising Standards Authority). Further guidance is provided by mental health service-user organisations or charitable groups such as Media Wise, which provides advice and guidance concerning media complaints. This process is vital as it might be argued that certain stigmatising images persist because of the lack of consumer feedback (Wahl 1995). Clearly, the outcome depends upon the credibility of the individual or organisation expressing dissatisfaction or the number of complaints received. This can have an almost instant response as can be seen with *The Sun* newspaper's withdrawal of their first edition coverage ('Bonkers Bruno') of Frank Bruno's hospitalisation for depression following a barrage of complaints.

The worst in media coverage is also showcased through Mind's annual *bigot of the year* awards with examples such as *The Sun*'s Paul Gilfeather and his article about Home Secretary Jack Straw's plans to introduce new powers of detention for people diagnosed with personality disorders with the headline of '600 Psychos to be Locked up'. The need for continued feedback concerning negative coverage is evidenced by the findings that the 'mentally ill' represent one of the most stigmatized conditions (Bloch and Singh 1997). They have traditionally been poorly protected unlike those in the categories of ethnic minorities, disabled and gender related who are supported through a wide range of legislation. It is therefore heartening to note the number of initiatives and campaigns (e.g. Mindshift and Changing Minds) that are currently helping to challenge the negative depiction of mental health themes and bring about a sense of change and optimism for the future.

Conclusion

To conclude this section, Berlo's model can be regarded as a cycle of communication with numerous factors and influences playing a core part through each stage of this process. People's attitudes and thoughts about mental health issues are not generated through a single cycle but can be regarded as the product of numerous revolutions with regard to a wide variety of media sources. It is a continuous process of bombardment by countless competing stimuli, carrying a full spectrum of messages both positive and negative. These issues are all addressed in depth within the following chapters which focus upon different media types and the influences and issues connected with them.

3   Stigma, labelling and the media: the negative representation of mental health issues

This chapter is concerned with the depiction within the media of negative stereotypes and stigmatising imagery relating to mental health issues. Negative representation is the predominant message being relayed and can be found in all media source types from the print media, film, TV and radio, through to the new electronic media. These negative messages are reinforced through countless examples which can be located both in historical and current media types. The degree to which stigmatising mental health imagery is reflected in the media is outlined in a number of current publications and reports such as the Mindout for Mental Health's (2001a) *Mindshift: a Guide to Open-Minded Coverage of Mental Health*, the Royal College of Psychiatrists' (2001) *Changing Minds: Every Family in the Land* and Mind's (2000) *Counting the Cost* report. These look at the extent of negative coverage of mental health issues and the effects upon the individual experiencing psychological problems. The significance of the predominantly negative portrayal is the maintenance and influence of stigmatising attitudes within societal and individuals' views. As Sieff (2003) identifies, the frequently negative frames deployed by the mass media contribute towards the persistence of the public's negative attitudes regarding the mentally ill. This sets up a cyclical relationship whereby negative perceptions are reinforced.

As identified by Bloch and Singh (1997), mental disorder and mental ill-health stand worldwide as being one of the most stigmatised of all human conditions. This is an alarming statement especially given the difficulty that may be experienced by many individuals within this group of representing themselves. There has been a shift over recent years towards a greater social awareness, enhanced advocacy and a greater 'voice' being developed (as well as perhaps permitted) regarding those experiencing mental health problems. This is complemented by campaigns and initiatives that promote positive mental health messages and challenge some of the commonly held myths and misrepresentations. Certainly with some stigmatised groups there has been a wealth of movement towards fostering a new culture of change and acceptance. The mentally ill have been left behind somewhat without the same level of sustained interest or concern and the negative representation of mental illness continues with representations that would be widely deemed as thoroughly unacceptable if associated with other marginalised groups. Indeed, as Wahl (1995) states, in the age of political correctness, people with mental illnesses are one of few remaining groups to be subject to such consistently thoughtless labelling. This process reflects the insidious and perpetuating nature of stigma whereby certain negative strands and assumptions are continuously reinforced.

As a starting place it is worth looking at definitions of stigma, defined by *The Oxford English Dictionary* as: 'A mark of disgrace or infamy; a sign of severe censure or condemnation, regarded as impressed on a person or thing; *a brand*' (*Oxford English Dictionary* 2005). A number of words stand out from this definition. First, those of *mark* and *brand* which both indicate some kind of distinguishing feature highlighting a sense of difference between the individual and others within their wider societal group. It is something which is easily identifiable and categorises the stigmatised as, to use Wahl's (1995) words, 'a breed apart'. It is interesting to note the origin of the term stigma, which related to a physical mark or brand made on Greek slaves to prevent their running away. It is perhaps this word *brand*, which more clearly evokes a sense of mental illness as a product of societal discrimination. It signifies an intentional process of creating some kind of mark that distinguishes the *mentally ill* from the *mentally well*. Individuals themselves may present with certain features that set them apart from others such as through what is observable by their appearance or behaviour. Whether these are deemed acceptable or not by various societal factions relates to the degree of stigmatising attitudes held by each specific group.

Another strand of the term stigma is the concept of labelling. As Becker (1963) stresses, once a label such as child molester or rapist is applied to someone, all actions that individual performs or has performed are interpreted in light of that label. Thomas Scheff (1974) proposed that the label *schizophrenic* activates stereotypes of mental illness learned in childhood from friends, family and the media. Certainly, mental illness references in children's media are common (Wilson *et al.* 2000) although are more often negative than positive with portrayals that typically disparage and ridicule (Wahl 2003a). An example from the *Beano* (16 August 2003) has the character Calamity James being chased around a park, first by a sabre wielding pirate ('Short John Saliva') and second by a First World War German pilot ('The Black Baron'). Their mentally ill status is made very clear both through their bizarre looks and violent behaviour, reinforced by Calamity James' final statement while running away: 'Waah! This park is chock full of loonies.' It is this type of exposure that leads us from an early age to see the mentally ill as being different.

One of the consequences of labelling is influencing the way in which people perceive themselves. Cooley's *The Looking Glass Self* stresses that one's identity and view of oneself is built primarily as a result of how others act and respond towards us (Cohen 1982). This is borne out by surveys such as Mind's (2000) *Counting the Cost* report which shows that individuals have had their self-esteem and confidence affected through negative media report-ing. While some people have the power to reject a negative label, many are unable to and therefore have to seek ways to cope with it (Becker 1963). This obviously presents potentially insurmountable obstacles for those who are already under-confident and psychologically vulnerable. Each label brings with it a set of expectations that foster responses such as dependence behaviour or accentuated eccentricity in those so categorised. Goffman (1963) refers to this process as *spurious interaction*, where the use of diag-nostic labels has a profoundly negative effect on the very behaviour of the patient. One such effect is the individual becoming in a sense a product of their label. This is reflected by Scheff (1974) and Kitwood (1997) with the view that an individual's illness behaviours are produced in part by the expectations placed upon them.

It is also worth noting that there is a negative effect on the behaviour of those people around them resulting in the labelled person being treated as 'sick' (Roediger *et al.* 1991). Once a person is labelled, professional carers will attach particular frames to an individual's conversation and actions. For example, a person's agitated behaviour might be regarded predominately as a result of their underlying psychopathology instead of their feelings of frus-tration or irritation at how powerless they are made to feel. This then picks up on other parts of the definition with words such as *condemnation* and *censure* that highlight the negative appeal and dismissive approach evoked. The term stigma has in common usage come to refer to any undesirable trait of an individual or group that devalues them and evokes negative or punitive responses (Susman 1994; Miles 1981). This view concurs with Goffman's (1963) view of stigma being socially discrediting, permanent and affecting the perception of the person as a whole. One issue here would relate to the identity of the person or group who does the branding, whether it is some-thing that is applied by society or the media. A common media response to criticism of its predominantly negative portrayal of mental illness is that it is merely reflecting the current picture in society, the brands therefore they would argue have already been applied.

One of the most commonly held misrepresentations is the association of violence and unpredictability with mental illness (Nairn *et al.* 2001; Wahl 1995). It is a representation that tends on the whole to be generalised more towards the psychotic disorders. Williams and Taylor (1995) report on a study that carried out a content analysis of 83 newspaper articles over a two-year period. The coverage was overly negative and reinforced the stereo-typical perception of the mentally ill as aggressive and unpredictable. Another study by Crisp *et al.* (2000) set out to determine the opinions of the British adult population (n = 1737) regarding their responses to seven types of mental disorder (severe depression, panic attacks, schizophrenia, dementia, eating disorders, alcoholism, drug addiction). The view that 'those with mental illness are dangerous' is held mostly with regard to schizo-phrenia, drug dependence and alcoholism. There was a widely held opinion that those experiencing mental health problems are hard to talk to, feel different from the way that we do and are unpredictable, which obviously accounts for some of the social distancing and isolation that is experienced.

Why do we stigmatise?

Wahl (1995) illustrates a number of potential reasons as to why such inaccurate representations of mental illness exist that include profit, ignorance, history, socialisation, psychological reassurance and lack of consumer feedback.

Profit

Profit provides a major incentive towards the continued use of stigmatising associations. As Salter and Byrne (2000) state, media is a business, its output driven by an overriding need to gain and sustain attention. It seems that the more dramatic the representation of *madness* the greater impact and selling potential it has. There is therefore a tendency among investors to repeat what has proved profitable in the past.

Ignorance

There is much that media personnel apparently do not know about mental illness. This is fuelled through common misconceptions held by members of the general public but are also shared by those working within media organisations. Recently, there have been attempts to challenge this through education of media personnel and liaison with professional or mental health service-user groups although many inaccurate and misrepresented portrayals continue to be used.

History

Images in today's mass media reflect conceptualisations and representations that have been around for centuries. This can be seen, for example, in the colloquial use of language that draws upon mental health terminology from a previous era, i.e. the regular featuring within tabloid headlines of words such as 'Lunatic' or 'Mental patient'. There are also representations that play upon the *possessed* theme evoking an earlier time where madness was seen as a visitation by divine forces.

Socialisation

The mass media can be regarded as the storytellers of today, acting as a primary socialising agent and passing on to their members the knowledge of the world. The significance here perhaps concerns which items out of the multitude available are selected and framed by media providers as being salient and appropriate for public consumption. Obviously, commercial considerations play a big part here and may result in fairly insignificant items being given a much higher priority than those having greater and farther-reaching consequences.

Psychological reassurance

Presenting the ill as different or dangerous may serve as a psychologically self-protective function. One reason is to do with predictability since being able to easily identify who is mentally ill means that members of the public can more easily take measures to protect themselves. There is also a polarisation process that takes place whereby the mentally ill are separated out and distanced from those who, by comparison, are deemed to be mentally well. The impression gained from many tabloid style depictions with their many stereotypes is that they are predominantly aimed at an audience who would wish to consider themselves as being mentally well.

Lack of consumer feedback

One of the historical problems resulting in the perpetuation of stigmatising portrayals has been the scarcity of feedback given to media providers. Another consideration is the weight or degree of reliability afforded those providing feedback, as more credibility is obviously afforded recognised groups over that of individuals. In recent years, though, campaigning and health promotion initiatives have meant that feedback about media depictions is taken on board far more strongly by those producing the various products on offer.

Maintaining stigma

It is interesting to consider factors that maintain the need for stigmatising or stereotypical representations. The need for media stereotypes can be seen as a way of presenting the receiver with reference points in what is experienced as a relentless stream of messages. As Valenti (2000) asserts, we are constantly bombarded by new information and stimuli and are not capable of an in-depth and instantaneous analysis of every aspect we encounter. The only way to manage this is through classifying and grouping according to familiar patterns. This is highlighted by Broadbent's (1958) filter theory which suggests we cope with a prolific amount of incoming stimuli by passing information through a filter. Haghighat (2001) looks at the pressure which the brain is under to respond to the proliferation of incoming stimuli and which copes with the increased demand by processing faster. He outlines that it may not therefore be as efficient to find out whether a person has qualities over and above what the name of their illness implies. This view is supported by

Rothbart *et al.* (1978) who indicate that when the brain is overloaded with data it is likely to treat examples of the behaviour of a single person as relatable to the behaviour of their group. Therefore examples of violence by mentally ill individuals tend to be generalised and transferred over to the wider grouping of those with mental health problems. Stigmatising messages therefore are pervasive, have lasting impact and devalue a lot of the mileage gained through campaigning and presentation of alternative, positive imagery. The greater impact from negative messages is indicated by the study of Kanouse and Hanson (1972) who have shown that the brain weights negative evaluations in preference to positive ones. The implications here are that positive health promotion and campaigning on their own are not enough and, for lasting change to occur, must be coupled with a dramatic reduction of negative and stigmatising presentations.

There are a number of factors which maintain the placing of the mentally ill as a group within a deviant category. One reinforcing aspect originates in societal intolerance and a fear of mental illness. This might transcend all attempts to educate the public as to the '*real*' facts concerning those with mental health problems and, for instance, their actual lower than expected potential for violence (DOH 1999). An interesting comparison is indicated by Laurance (2003) who points out that we actually show greater tolerance to what are much more lethal behaviours such as dangerous driving and alcohol abuse which are shown to kill or maim a larger number of people. This brings up the notion of societal *scapegoating*, with the mentally ill presenting easier targets on whom to visit all of our unwanted or negative feelings. It highlights Foucault's (1961) notion of madness being a constructed entity and something that we prefer to externalise onto others. The sense of distancing and separation shown here between the mentally well and the mentally ill is strongly found throughout the institutional era with the purging of *madness* from within families and society. It is a process that can also be found within therapeutic environments as shown by Kantor and Gelineau's (1965) study that observed staff members actually stimulating continued symptom expression among patients in subtle ways. Although they were not aware of this dynamic, the influences behind this behaviour were felt to be concerned with maintaining a clear and psychologically needed distinction between patient and helper. It is interesting therefore to note the view that deviance is not a quality of the act the person commits, but rather a consequence of the application by others of rules and sanctions (Becker 1963).

Clearly one of the main reasons for the inclusion of stigmatising and stereotypical mental health portrayals by the media is the dramatic impact that they have upon their audience. This results in aspects regarding the mentally ill often being distorted and exaggerated in order to make products more appealing to their audience (Nunnally 1981). Despite some very detailed sets of guidelines concerning media content (i.e. the Broadcasting Standards Commission 1998; Independent Television Commission 2002; and the National Union of Journalists 1999), it seems that in many cases the advice given is ignored in favour of a sensational or eye-catching approach. It is evident that madness as a topic is very commercially appealing and that this in many cases overrides the degree of sensitivity being shown to those who are stigmatised.

The effects of stigma

The most impactful factors affecting those who are stigmatised concerns an individual's critical self-perception as well as the distancing and rejecting response experienced from others. Stigma therefore can be seen as a process that is either generated from a process of internal or external feedback (see Figure 3.1). These elements are echoed in Scambler's (1998) aspects of stigma concerning felt stigma and enacted stigma.

Felt stigma (internal stigma)

The frequent bombardment of derogatory language such as 'mentals', 'nutters', 'lunatics' and 'psycho', as well as the frequent use of unflattering and unrealistic imagery cannot help to engender good feelings in those with mental health problems. The first issue here is the felt experience and the issue of self-stigmatisation concerning how individuals come to reappraise their experience in light of media coverage. This is illustrated by Gilbert (2003) with regard to the process of external and internal shame. The *external* shame might include the feeling that 'others see me as unattractive' which results in a sense of *internal* shame in that 'I see myself as unattractive'. The shame and

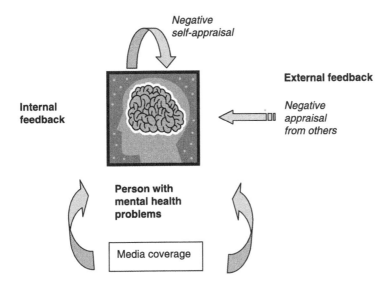

Figure 3.1 Stigma and negative appraisal.

expectation of discrimination prevents people from talking about their experiences and discourages them from seeking help. An individual's concept of self is affected through stigma with enhanced feelings of hopelessness, low self-worth and increased social withdrawal (Gray 2002). The prejudice and discrimination experienced can compound the distress felt and interfere further with personal coping skills already affected as a result of mental health problems (Johnstone 2001). These features are all reflected in Mind's (2000) *Counting the Cost* report which details the negative impact that media coverage has upon those experiencing mental health problems. The cycle of disadvantage is illustrated by the Social Exclusion Unit (2003) in that once mental health problems develop, they can often have a negative impact on employability, housing, income and opportunities to access services and social networks, potentially leading to severe economic deprivation and social isolation. Indeed, studies conducted in the late 1990s illustrate that only 13 per cent of those with long-term mental health problems were actually working compared to 35 per cent among the physically disabled (Sayce 2000). As is stressed by Link *et al.* (2001), a major consequence of reducing stigma is to improve the self-esteem of those with mental illnesses. It is worth mentioning, however, that not all of those who are stigmatised will be unable to respond or cope with the deluge of negative imagery and representations in the media. This is illustrated in Camp *et al.*'s (2002) study of women with chronic mental health problems who, although being aware of societal responses and attitudes and the effects it had on their lives, did not accept these representations as valid and rejected them as applicable to themselves.

A number of those experiencing mental health problems indicate the extreme feelings of anxiety felt regarding their 'coming out'. As Sayce (2000) states, for some this can be a liberating experience yet for others it can be hard to reconcile the different aspects of themselves such as competent researcher and mental health survivor. Certainly, the liberating process is reflected upon in a number of autobiographical accounts, as demonstrated by the footballer Tony Adams writing in the book *Addicted* about his coping with alcoholism. The 'coming out' by notable individuals is in some cases greeted favourably by the public as exampled by Norwegian Prime Minister Mr Bondevik's decision to take time off with depression, an action applauded by the public and even his political opponents. Another notable example was the revelation by Princess Diana about her struggles with the eating disorder bulimia. The importance of sharing such experiences publicly cannot be overestimated as it means that the taboo surrounding certain mental health states is reduced and the featured condition is afforded degrees of acceptance, thereby facilitating others talking about and sharing related issues. This all plays a major role in reducing the sense and feeling of felt stigma experienced by those with mental health problems.

Enacted stigma (external stigma)

Essentially what stereotypical and stigmatising portrayals do is to objectify and distance those with mental illness from others in society. A large percentage of media portrayals tend to offer us representations of mental illness which show little regard for the actual person and their felt experience. The predominant perspective is one that outlines the potential threat posed to the rest of society by those deemed to be mentally unfit. Responsibility for perpetuating stereotypes is to a large extent attributed to the media, although this is largely rejected with the claim that they are merely mirroring the values and beliefs held already within society (Bolton 2000). The origin of stigma is a topic that evokes considerable debate although it can certainly be regarded as a cyclical process whereby both societal attitudes and media portrayals strongly influence each other. This can be reflected in the view that what we learn about mental health issues is largely generated by what is picked up from the media (Philo 1996a). The media subsequently develop products that are regarded as appealing and reflecting the needs and interests of their audience.

A major problem affecting the mentally ill through the process of stigmatisation is that of social exclusion, which this is well documented in a number of studies such as Mind's (2000) *Counting the Cost* report and the Social Exclusion Unit's (2003) project. Recent attempts to tackle this include the setting up of the Social Exclusion Unit, which initiated a project in 2003 to tackle the barriers to opportunity faced by adults with mental health problems. This is a governmental initiative with the core aims of investigating what can be done to enable more adults with mental health problems to enter and to retain work, as well as having the same opportunities for social participation and access to services as the general population. Such schemes are vital in helping tackle both the impact upon the person with mental health problems as well as the rejecting and distancing attitudes held by others towards them. These attitudes have also been noted with regard to care delivery where services are driven to some degree by fear and where risk reduction through containment is the norm. At the same time that mental health service-users are calling for greater empowerment and autonomy, care services are responding with an authoritarian risk-reduction approach (Laurance 2003). This has in part been influenced by media coverage of well publicised incidents of homicides, violence and suicide where policy measures which have been introduced in response to public concerns have only served to impose additional constraints on those with mental health problems (Hallam 2002). It fits in with Linné and Warfella's (1998) view of *moral panics*, the effects that are supposed to emerge when the media consistently represent a subgroup or subculture as being dangerous or deviant.

Courtesy stigma

The power of stigma is such that it does not reside alone with the mentally ill but can be widened to include others such as families, friends and carers (Östman and Kjellin 2002). Stigma by association or 'courtesy stigma' relates to the problems whereby the family of a 'mentally ill' individual may share some of the discredit of their stigmatised relative (Angermeyer *et al.* 2003). This then widens the example to encompass the family as a dysfunctional unit and to some degree explains the desire by some family groups to safeguard their own interests by 'expelling' the sick member. The aspect of how stigma affects and envelops others close to and involved with the mentally ill has been paid little attention by researchers. The concept of family burden has been looked at although not specifically with regards to the concept of stigma. Wally Lamb's fictional novel, *I Know This Much is True*, provides a vivid account of the impact that mental illness has on other members of the family. This book centres upon Thomas's experience of schizophrenia and the psychological suffering and burden of guilt endured by both his twin brother Dominick and his stepfather Ray. It is a powerful narrative that highlights the need to understand how mental health issues and associated stigma affects family members and their subsequent requirements from psychiatric services.

The concept of courtesy stigma can also be widened to encompass those treating the mentally ill. This is particularly illustrated within the cinema through numerous films depicting the professional carers every bit as, if not more, disturbed than those they are treating (Clare 2001). One of the messages being portrayed here, as conveyed very strongly through the film *Shock Corridor*, is of contamination through becoming too intimately involved with madness. Another aspect concerns the attractiveness of the psychiatric professions to psychologically disturbed individuals, as with the murderous psychiatrists Hannibal Lecter in *The Silence of the Lambs* and Dr Robert Elliot in *Dressed to Kill*. It is certainly alarming to witness such depictions involving those we place our trust in when at our most vulnerable.

What's bad about . . .?

This section focuses upon a selection of media types and features some of the more prominently negative characteristics or examples portrayed. The sources covered are those of film, TV, Internet, press and literature.

. . . Film

Characterisation

A character's appearance conveys some very strong messages to the audience. From a mental health perspective numerous stereotypes are employed whereby selected individuals are framed through their looks, speech or behaviour as being different. There may be a fair degree of deliberation in the casting of characters that fit some of the typical notions as to what the mentally ill look like. An example here can be seen in the typecasting of Peter Lorre who, because of his distinctively odd appearance, was chosen to play the deranged killer in a succession of films. Their portrayal is often aided by a number of accompanying cues, which highlight factors such as the dangerousness of the character (Hannibal Lecter's wildly excessive collection of restraints), a person's social ineptitude (Geoffrey Rush's dishevelled portrayal of David Helfgott in *Shine*) or the wide gulf between wellness and illness (Jim Carrey's Jekyll and Hyde portrayal in *Me, Myself and Irene*). These characterisations help to perpetuate the societal myth that we can spot those with mental health problems by their appearance and behaviour alone. It serves to further distance those with mental health problems from others and fits Wahl's (1995) classification of 'a breed apart'.

The mentally ill as killers

The stereotypical association between violence and mental health issues is found in prolific quantity within the medium of film. The imagery provided by the showcasing of the mentally ill killer provides the viewer with a heightened sense of tension, drama and excitement. In a number of cases, these types of film also meet individuals' needs for catharthis and curiosity regarding what violent impulses look like (Wolfenstein and Leites 1970). Films within this genre are enormously appealing to audiences and sometimes even receive critical acclaim, factors that help to ensure their continued appearance (Wahl 1995). A major problem with this is the maintenance of the association between mental illness and a person's propensity for violence, leaving the receiver with a feeling of unease and disquiet (Byrne 2001a). These powerful stereotypical messages undermine attempts made at educating the public through various campaigns and health promotion initiatives. The related imagery and language are so pervasive and have permeated our culture to such a degree that words such as '*psycho*' have come to represent homicidal impulses or an unpredictable and deranged mind (Welch and Racine 1999). The peculiar establishment of some of the murderous characters who are featured as cult heroes (such as Hannibal Lecter and Freddy Krueger) only serves to establish the link more fully within our subconscious.

Misrepresentation

A key feature evoking criticism about film portrayals of mental illness relates to the huge number of inaccuracies or misrepresentations being shown. One film in particular that was greeted with a fair amount of critical rebuke for its offensively inaccurate portrayal is that of *Me, Myself and Irene*. This movie erroneously featured the main character's split personality with the good self being manifested in his mentally well part and the bad self represented by his mentally ill one. The fact that this film proved such a huge success at the box office is a depressing one given the number of people exposed to such negative and misleading facts about mental illness. The scale of misrepresentation within the cinema is huge and even extends towards the 'based upon a true story' type of film. For example, David Helfgott's sister Margaret stressed that her father and the hospital staff treating her brother were not as harsh or oppressive as their portrayal in the film *Shine* suggested (Rosen and Walter 2000). This was clearly built up and exaggerated for the benefit of offering the viewer cues for dramatic engagement. Another example is the film *A Beautiful Mind* which can be regarded as misrepresentative by its omission of certain facts, such as Nash's younger son's diagnosis of schizophrenia, an issue strongly featured within Sylvia Nasar's (1998) biographical work. It is certainly true that condensing a person's life story down into about ninety minutes of film is obviously going to be a difficult task. It may involve over-dramatising certain elements in order to engage and stir the emotions of the audience but it also means that, because of available space, certain features are omitted. The story presented to the audience therefore can be regarded as a construct of the director, scriptwriter and film crew, with commercial and artistic considerations having a major say in how the person's story is told.

... TV

Dramatic licence

As within the cinema, there are many examples whereby those with mental health problems are grossly misrepresented. This was noted in particular by Wilson *et al.*'s (1999) study of prime time television dramas that found a predominantly negative characterisation of mentally ill characters being used. This saw them being depicted as dangerous, simple, unpredictable and socially inept. These examples feature strongly within the hospital dramas and *Holby City* and *Casualty* in particular regularly carry storylines where mentally disturbed characters add an extra spice to the drama being served up. For instance, *Holby City* carried a storyline reminiscent of the Beverly Allitt case with a nurse killing some of her patients. Some clues were given as to the causes of this nurse's psychological disturbance although providing the viewer with another portrayal that associated the concepts of 'mentally ill' and 'dangerous'. The addition of mentally ill characters also occurs in soaps where enhanced audience engagement is desired. It is not coincidental that in many of these cases the television ratings are enhanced. This is particularly true in the case of psychopathically disturbed individuals such as 'Mad Maya' in *Coronation Street* or Sarah in *Eastenders*. It is clearly the case that madness is attractive to viewers and certainly something that adds extra drama or impact to products.

Exploitation

This section relates primarily to the increasingly popular genres of the chat show and reality TV formats. The chat shows range from the sensitive and informative to the grossly exploitative and abusive. The former include shows such as *Esther* and to some degree *Oprah*, which feature some important social issues (i.e. abuse and bereavement) and treat their participants with a degree of respect and sensitivity. There is also an important function here for viewers who can engage in a form of vicarious therapy, connecting with and feeling supported by the experience shared by participants. The latter, though, include examples (such as *Trisha* and J*erry Springer*) where the needs of participants appear to be relegated behind those of providing the audience with an entertaining show. The feeling here is of individuals being deliberately manipulated by the charismatic facilitator towards confrontational situations and displays of distress or anger, the stronger the emotion, it seems, the better. The sense of individuals 'performing' for the audience's pleasure is very strongly conveyed through the numerous *reality TV* shows that dominate our viewing schedules. Some are loosely packaged along the social experiment lines reminiscent of studies such as Zimbardo's 1971 Stanford University prison experiment which placed volunteers in the roles of prisoners and guards. The experiment had to be stopped after six out of the planned fourteen days because of the pathological reactions being displayed by most of the participants, five of whom were released earlier than planned because of depression (Haney and Zimbardo 1998). This then raises an important issue concerning the increasing lack of concern being shown towards those participating within television shows as viewers are regularly entertained by a person's public humiliation or abuse. The lack of respect for participants is also to some degree shared by the audience, illustrated by the level of celebration afforded those involved in abusing others such as *Pop Idol*'s Simon Cowell. It is also reflected in the high viewing figures with shows featuring the abuse of contestants proving very popular, for example the jungle contest *I'm a Celebrity Get Me Out of Here* had various trials where contestants were bitten by snakes, covered in spiders or viciously pecked by emus. All of this aptly sums up Woods' (2002) statement about reality TV as a form of mass voyeurism where a person's dignity no longer matters.

. . . The Internet

Information overload

One of the biggest strengths of the Internet also provides one of its main problems in that the easy availability and access of vast stores of information causes problems for consumers in terms of sifting through and selecting what is relevant. The almost limitless amount of material retrievable means that those searching the Internet are faced with an overload of information

(Christensen and Griffiths 2000). As Cooke (2001) indicates, this problem is compounded by the way in which many search tools are programmed to retrieve as much as possible of the available material. This poses significant problems in selecting out what is pertinent as well as having the time and ability to process it. Some of these aspects are highlighted by Scrivener (2002) as the mistaking of unrefined data for knowledge; the stockpiling of information; and the failure to appraise information through time mismanagement. This all means that some of the valid and worthy material accessible online remains unseen or unappreciated by many of those at whom it is targeted.

Confusing or harmful material

A brief search of the Internet can prove a bewildering and confusing process as a fair degree of the information accessed appears contrary to that found on other more authoritative sites. Mixed in with all of the educative and supportive health sites are some that can be extremely misleading and harmful. In some cases Internet sites post erroneous material as a result of ignorance or a lack of understanding concerning the aspects being relayed. In other cases poorly evidenced information is very deliberately included for an individual or a group's personal reasons. Their agenda here is not always clear although might be borne out of an individual's own dissatisfying experience of health care. This would in some instances explain the posting within anti-psychiatry sites of information such as 'All psychiatric drugs are harmful'. In most cases no credible evidence is given to support wildly subjective claims such as this and it is common to find information being provided mostly through personal rhetoric. As Thompson (1999) indicates, a major concern relates to the uncertain type of information that desperate people might be exposed to. It is therefore very worrying to reflect upon those Internet sites which advocate self-harmful behaviours and sanitise the very real and distressing nature of suicide through their use of terms such as 'self-deliverance'.

... The press

Misinformation

Given that we learn a large percentage of our information from the media, it is perhaps disturbing to consider the degree to which we are actually being misinformed. The reliability of what we are exposed to varies significantly and news can be regarded either as a reflection of what is occurring in society or as a construction by journalists (Potter 2004). Reporting styles have come under much scrutiny over the years and it is interesting to note a Media Bureau (2001) study which indicates that a large percentage (64 per cent) of reporters themselves believe that the coverage of news should be better. The degree to which misleading items are down to the journalists' lack of knowledge or due to the pressures to present a more commercially appealing product is unclear.

One of the most frequently portrayed categories when writing about the mentally ill concerns that of violent behaviour (Philo *et al.* 1996; Nairn *et al.* 2001). Although this association is strongly contended by a wealth of evidence suggesting that the mentally ill present a low risk of harming others (DOH 1999), it continues to be reinforced by many subjective and poorly constructed news items. A more dramatic style of reporting is clearly attractive to readers and helps, despite the various regulations applicable, to maintain poor and misleading journalistic styles.

Stigmatisation

The main thread here is of a negative depiction primarily through words but also to some extent through associated imagery. The public are treated on a regular basis to many examples where stories are presented in sensationalist style with many phrases or words such as 'mental patient', 'psycho killer' or 'patient escaped' being used for dramatic effect. These terms stand out forcibly from the background and are often attached to other well-recognised aspects to heighten their effect, such as '*Silence of the Lambs* Maniac Freed to Kill'. The association with a person's violence potential is complemented by other negative portrayals such as that of mental deficiency or powerlessness. The main types of characterisation used, therefore, are either geared towards evoking feelings of unease and discomfort or those of pity and paternalism. Both of these are stigmatising reactions which place the other person at a distance from us and do not encourage acceptance or empowerment. The three main ingredients for a 'top story', as highlighted by Kalbfleisch (1979), were insanity, unpredictability and victimisation of ordinary people. Clearly, the perpetuation of insensitive and stigmatising depictions is strongly influenced by the fact that they help publications to sell.

Contradictions

There are many examples that can be found within the print media where conflicting or ambiguous messages are presented. This occurs frequently in most of the glossy magazines which showcase and promote various health issues such as stress, body image and eating disorders. While on its own this is laudable enough, in many cases there is a fair degree of competition from conflicting stimuli in the form of pictures and features which pursue perfection or mercilessly expose and attack imperfection through 'Caught on Camera' type features. The newsprint media is an extremely effective channel for conveying health promotion because of its exposure potential and readership by large numbers of people. In a number of cases, though, the potential benefits are outweighed and somewhat confused by the contradictory messages also being relayed. A prime example of this is *The Sun* newspaper's sudden shift towards mental health campaigner in the wake of the widespread criticism and condemnation following their appalling 'Bonkers Bruno' headlines. However, this did not deter the newspaper from continuing to display less than flattering or ridiculing messages such as the picture of Frank Bruno in pantomime costume.

... *Literature*

Destructiveness to self

There are a number of publications that feature mental illness as a destructive entity with regard to self. This type of writing follows an individual's gradual fragmentation and eventual consumption through their mental health state. A notable example here is that of Malcolm Lowry's *Under the Volcano* depicting the ex-consul Geoffrey Firmin's gradual alienation and destruction through alcoholism. A particular issue is the portrayal of the protagonist as powerless and unable to do much about slowing down or preventing their eventual fate. It also features the helplessness of others who are unable to provide sufficient support. One factor worth highlighting here is the stage in a person's illness when the narrative is written. The book *Catcher in the Rye* features Holden Caulfield's deteriorating mental health state and finishes the narrative with his future progression uncertain. An interesting comparison can be provided through autobiographical accounts that take the reader beyond the time of crisis towards a place of resolution and hope. Without the 'happy ending', stereotypes such as mental illness as an unrecoverable state, are fostered.

Destructiveness to others

The other type of depiction focuses on the destructive potential towards others and can be found within the extremely popular genre of psycho-killer fiction (e.g. Patricia Cornwell's *Body of Evidence* or Ian McEwan's *Enduring Love*). The essence of this type of writing is the placing of the 'mad murderer' as an external threat to the mentally well heroic central figures. This provides the reader with a touch of drama and engagement with the text although again serves to reinforce a negative misassumption concerning mental illness. Another issue is the location of the mentally ill as a destructive or controlling presence in the background. Books such as *Jane Eyre* (Mrs Rochester) and *Cold Comfort Farm* (Aunt Ada) feature characters who, despite being rarely seen, hold a strong controlling influence over central characters. This again promotes mental illness very much in a negative and destructive light.

Negative representations of mental illness

The following section identifies some of the core themes running throughout much of this work where negative representations of mental illness are fostered. These include aspects where the mentally ill are characterised as being different, the power or language, other related prejudices and images of perfection.

The mentally ill as 'a breed apart'

A predominant feature, as briefly alluded to earlier in the allocation of stigma, is the perception of difference, or as Wahl (1995) determines, identifying the mentally ill as 'a breed apart'. According to a large majority of media portrayals, the mentally ill are portrayed as looking different and acting peculiarly, thereby separating them from what are seen as the 'normal' population. It serves a function of making them easily identifiable and to some degree, as far as the general public is concerned, controllable. These types of representation leave the receiver in little doubt as to which of all the characters shown to them have altered mental health states. *Difference* is made to stand out forcibly and is therefore more readily noticeable as with the Gestalt concept of figure and ground (King and Wertheimer 2005). A predisposition to notice difference is something that is innate to all human (and many animal) groups, since they depend upon the predictable behaviour of their members for their functioning and safety (Smith 2002). However, it is worth clarifying the point that difference can to a large extent be imagined, exaggerated or applied according to one's expectations, as is often the case with regard to mental illness. The characterisation and portrayal of distinct differences in a number of cases makes mental illness a visible entity either through imagery, narrative or terminology. The exaggerated physical characteristics, dramatic and unpredictable behaviour and asocial lifestyles have come to represent what might be regarded as the uniform of the mentally ill. For instance, *Schizophrenic* the debut album by JC Chasez not very imaginatively features the singer in a straight jacket on its cover.

The two core strands of observable difference can be seen as *Looks* and *Behaviour* with the mentally ill being shown to appear and act in ways which signify their altered mental health state. In a number of stereotypical examples, the mentally ill are portrayed as bizarre, ghoulish or deformed. This includes at times a deliberate casting of individuals who are sufficiently 'weird' or 'odd' looking (e.g. Peter Lorre). It also involves those whose screen behaviour and demeanour seem well suited for the part, for instance Jim Carrey in the film *Me, Myself and Irene*. Perhaps over time the extent of exaggeration with regard to visible characteristics has been toned down although is still prominently visible within genres such as horror films or children's television. The horror film incorporates many of the classic stereotypes leaving us in no doubt as to the sense of threat presented by the psychopathic killer, who clearly *looks* dangerous. Even when the killer's physical appearance appears fairly normal, accompanying cues are used to exemplify traits and aspects which we might not otherwise see. For example, the excessive use of restraint used to transport Hannibal Lecter clearly signifies the degree of danger which is present despite any reassurances of safety given.

The portrayal of difference is also prolifically found within children's media and in particular television programmes with the predominant representation of mental illness featuring exaggerated physical attributes and behaviours (Wilson *et al.* 2000). These portrayals present children with a distorted view of the world as well as having a significant impact upon their subsequent attitudes and beliefs (Vooijs and Van der Voort 1993). This theme is not limited to the visible medium and can be found in abundance within the newsprint media and the world of literature where words are used to convey ways in which the mentally ill present as being different. Charlotte Brontë's *Jane Eyre* for example provides a clear example of this with Mrs Rochester being portrayed more as a wild beast than a human being. There are certainly numerous examples to be found within the tabloid press where the violent or socially inadequate mentally ill stereotypes are heavily featured.

It seems that the mentally ill within much of the media are destined to be presented as looking or behaving according to what is expected of them. There have over the past few years been a number of notable attempts to change this and provide media consumers with less stereotypical and more realistic representations. For example, the portrayal of Zoe Tate's schizo-phrenic breakdown in *Emmerdale* has been covered generally with a greater degree of sensitivity and compassion than most other depictions. The typical representation of mental illness on television generally characterises the individual as violent, bad, a victim or a failure (Signorielli 1989). In contrast to this, the *Emmerdale* example featured a character who was a wealthy businesswoman and successful veterinary surgeon as well as being likeable and fundamentally good. It was disappointing therefore to note the occasions on which her character reverted to stereotype with scenes such as the setting fire to a church, barricading her children in the kitchen of her house or her apparent involvement in the near killing of her daughter's father. Programme makers perhaps have found it too difficult to resist the dramatic potential presented by her illness.

Language and terminology

When debating what is acceptable and what isn't concerning the presentation of mental health themes, we need to view them in the context within which they are presented. First, we have the notion of historical applicability where it can be seen that what is deemed acceptable or unacceptable is forever changing. Indeed, the terminology used in conjunction with mental illness strongly indicates this. An example relates to the language used to denote those who are mentally ill ranging from terms such as *lunatics, mentally deficient, mentally ill,* through to some of the currently used titles such as *mental health service-users* in the UK or *survivors* and *consumers* in the US. Equally, the setting within which care is delivered has also been subject to a wide range of definitions including *madhouse, lunatic asylum, psychiatric hospital* and *mental health unit.* Clearly, many other terms could be added to this list including those used jargonistically or offensively within the media but which have subsequently become fairly mainstream words, for example *psycho* or *mental home*. Whether or not changing terminology does anything to combat stigmatising attitudes is debatable. Often, the wording that was acceptable in a previous era (e.g. *lunatic*) signifies a lack of understanding and care when used in the present context. It is a process highlighted by Haghighat (2001) with regard to the language used within legislation and learning difficulties, each term acquiring the discrediting connotations of the previous one. It is evident that the single approach of changing terminology does little to combat the overall effects of stigmatisation of the mentally ill and that a much more concerted educative and health promotional approach is required.

It is clear that words influence our relationship and feelings towards those with mental health problems. The widespread and prolific use of disparaging terms within the media helps to foster an 'us and them' dynamic. It is very much a distancing process which diminishes the opportunities for actual connection and appreciation of another person's felt experience. The stigmatising power of words is reflected by Sartorius (2002), who highlights in particular the careless use of diagnostic labels. The common misuse of certain terms means that they will be adopted and used more widely by others who do not realise the errors being made. A common misrepresentation is the interchangeable use made of certain terms that includes the association of schizophrenia with that of 'split personality'. Other interchangeably misused terms include those of 'psychotic' and 'psychopathic' as well as 'learning difficulties' and 'mental illness' (Wahl 1995). The exposure to careless, stigmatising and inaccurate references permeates the whole of the media and starts at a very young age. As Wilson *et al.* (2000) worryingly found, there are countless 'mental illness' references being made even within children's media with the vocabulary including many negative and derogatory terms such as 'crazy', 'mad', 'losing your mind', 'wacko', 'cuckoo' and 'loony'.

Pictures of perfection

There are a number of other ways in which negative messages regarding mental illness are conveyed other than the more obvious stigmatising portrayals. It might include media products where positive messages are notably absent or indeed those which 'sell' images of *perfection*. These are found prolifically within large sections of the media and in particular on television and within magazines. The need to address this issue is reflected by the findings that prolonged exposure to images of perfection can have a significantly negative impact upon those receiving them (Durkin 2002; Martinez-Gonzalez *et al.* 2003). The popularity of these types of media product has been noted by a number of sources, and women's magazines in particular attain high levels of exposure with circulation rates in some instances running into millions (Borman 2003).

The overly attentive focus upon beauty issues and the strong conveyance of flawless images all help to draw attention towards the opposite position, that of imperfection. The implications here are that not looking a certain way is subsequently felt as unacceptable and lowers a person's tolerance towards any type of 'flaw'. The huge selling of perfection is complemented by an almost smug, gloating approach which can be found where certain types of imperfection are spotted, for example when celebrities dare to be casually dressed or even worse perhaps display signs of fat. In these cases, any perceived flaw identified is mercilessly and insensitively treated. The choice of words used also compounds this problem with commonly used terms such as 'perfect' regularly found at one end of the spectrum compared to a range of disparaging and insensitive ones being reflected at the other end. For example, *Now* magazine's 'Exclusive Caught on Camera Feature' includes a collection of unflattering pictures of the television presenter Eammon Holmes leaving a cake shop with captions such as 'Laden with an overflowing bag of goodies he can't wait to get home and tuck in'. This ridiculing and abusive approach centres primarily upon his weight and appearance, engaging readers in having a laugh at his expense. It is an extremely insensitive and offensive approach although more accepted by publishers and readers with celebrities being regarded as 'fair game'. The major problem, though, is the impact that these approaches have upon the general population where beauty is venerated and imperfection is regarded as intolerable. It is made worse by the increase of methods to help people in their pursuit of looking younger and more attractive. Magazines frequently carry advertising offering products and treatments such as cosmetic surgery and liposuction. The need to resort to some of these methods is stimulated further by a host of television programmes demonstrating the 'marvellous' transformation from frumpy to attractive before our eyes. This is achieved through a number of methods such as rigorous dieting, hairdressing, make-up, clothing, as well as certain surgical techniques. We are also shown the humiliating and demeaning processes that participants go through as they are manipulated towards change in a very forthright and critical fashion. For example, in *What Not to Wear*, Trinny and Susannah maintain a running commentary on the featured person's appearance letting them know in no uncertain terms if they are making a poor choice with regard to what they are wearing. This all appears fairly mild when compared to shows such as *10 Years Younger* where the treatment of the participant is often offensive and humiliating, being paraded in front of the public by the presenter Nicky Hambleton-Jones in order to initially receive some insulting and critical comments. The purpose of this is for the viewer's benefit to help achieve a feeling of before and after contrast with the subsequent parading in front of the public evoking more complimentary noises and comments. The process of transition though is a harsh one involving invasive physical treatments such as chemical peels and nose surgery. It is interesting therefore to consider the thoughts of the average television viewer who is unable to attain such a transformation because of financial or other reasons. There is certainly evidence to suggest that exposure to these types of media messages has a detrimental effect upon many people's concept of self and to some degree helps to explain the dramatic uptake in cosmetic surgery over recent years (Wykes and Gunter 2005). Until the message being sent out by the media becomes more balanced, the need by many to strive towards an unattainable goal will be maintained.

Associated prejudice

The sense of stigma may be further heightened when mental illness is linked with other groups which are also marginalised for reasons of race, gender and disability. An alarming consequence of this can be seen in the higher incidence of Afro-Caribbean individuals than expected entering the psychiatric in-patient system (McGovern and Cope 1987) or being diagnosed with schizophrenia at a rate 12–13 times higher than the average number (Harrison *et al.* 1988). As Weiss *et al.* (2001) point out, an understanding of what stigma means involves looking at how it is viewed across cultures as it is not evident that different cultures will regard the same features as salient with regard to stigma.

Negative representations of those with mental health problems are compounded by prejudicial attitudes such as those of a racial nature. In some instances, the reporting of black people with mental health problems uses descriptions or terms which do not adequately reflect the person being reported. Certain descriptors stand out very forcibly and in a sense are used representatively to highlight the essence of the person being reported and to draw us as readers into a particular relationship with them. For example, if we consider headlines such as 'Mum Attacked by Black Mental Patient', we have a way of relating immediately to the subjects contained within the article. Without reading any further, we can feel a sense of pity towards the victim ('mum'), an adverb that signifies qualities of kindness, caring and nurturing. On the other hand, the 'Black Mental Patient' is used to convey a sense of threat, complemented by the commonly applied reading of 'big, black and dangerous'. What these types of portrayals do is to depersonalise the individual and reduce them to a collection of catch phrases. It is a point reflected by Wilson (1997) who states that when newspapers turn a black man who has committed a violent crime into a 'psycho killer', 'schizophrenic killer', or 'Beast of Belgravia', they endlessly obliterate the person behind the label.

It is interesting, therefore, to note the National Union of Journalist's (1999) *Code of Conduct* Clause 10 which affirms that:

A journalist shall only mention a person's race, colour, creed, illegitimacy, marital status (or lack of it), gender or sexual orientation if this information is strictly relevant. A journalist shall neither originate nor process material which encourages discrimination, ridicule, prejudice or hatred on any of the above-mentioned grounds.

(NUJ 1999)

Instead of adhering to this code, there is at times an almost blatant disregard shown to individuals or groups of people through the references which are made. Numerous adjectives have been used to describe a person experiencing mental health problems, many of them far from flattering. One of the core problems with prejudicial and discriminatory attitudes is the sense of marginalisation and distance created between separate groups. As illustrated by Van Dijk (1987) these negative views are kept alive by the central role that these beliefs play in the symbolic world of the majority, allowing them to form a comfortable in-group identity. In this instance, negative associations are applied to the stigmatised groups and externalised from those who deem themselves to be mentally well.

Tackling stigma

Corrigan and Penn (1999) suggest three basic ways in which groups can confront stigma – through 'Protest', 'Education' and 'Contact'. These issues are covered in more detail in the following chapter although will be briefly addressed here.

Protest

Priebe (2003) confirms the picture that efforts to achieve more positive attitudes are operating within the background of a predominantly negative coverage of mental health issues. Changing attitudes or confirming positive stereotypes according to Rothbart and Park (1986) requires a larger number of positive examples and fewer contrary examples to disconfirm it. It also needs a sustained level of critical feedback concerning portrayals that are less than accurate or flattering. Over the past few years a number of organisations representing governmental, heath professional and service-user groups have become very active in campaigning against stigmatising coverage of mental health issues in the media. Critical feedback to media providers about their coverage linked with education and guidance has helped to reduce some of the stereotypical content found across all media types. It appears though that the response to protest is exceedingly slow and perhaps instances of change and response are due in large part to worries over the potential commercial implications. This was highlighted strongly with *The Sun* newspapers surprising U-turn with regard to their coverage of the Frank Bruno story from insensitive and stigmatising to staunch mental health advocate.

Education

While often perpetrating negative stereotypes, if properly harnessed the media may be used to combat stigma (Salter and Byrne 2000). Crisp *et al.*'s (2000) study found that in most instances stigmatising opinions are based upon factors other than a general lack of knowledge about mental disorder. It follows here that destigmatising campaigns have to do more than simply educate and increase knowledge. This viewpoint is shared by Haghighat (2001) who indicates that people need more than logic, as providing rational evidence that refutes a schizophrenic individual's propensity for violence does not necessarily combat their already conditioned autonomic circuit of arousal, fear and anxiety. This reflects Bodenhausen's (1993) findings that it is the feeling rather than the cognitive component of attitudes that determines people's social judgement. Destigmatising approaches therefore clearly need to address the emotional content and enable people with means of ventilating and understanding associated anxiety.

Contact

The importance of contact with the mentally ill as a destigmatising approach is also outlined by Penn *et al.* (1994). This helps individuals to appreciate something of the reality experienced by people with mental illness, thereby countering many stereotypical notions. A degree of contact is also provided through media examples such as autobiographical accounts and television documentaries which highlight the actual lived and felt experience of mental illness. For example, the documentary programme *Inside my Head: Michael* featured a 16-year-old boy with two severe schizophrenia episodes already behind him. His frank and exposing honesty in the face of abuse and worsening symptoms provided the viewer with a strong opportunity for connection and understanding of the condition of schizophrenia. These types of example importantly foster connecting and empathic approaches, something sadly lacking in the majority of media depictions.

4 Selling mental health (positive health promotion)

Introduction

As has been illustrated in the previous chapter, there is a predominantly negative portrayal of mental health issues to be found within the media as a whole. This is illustrated through various reports and studies that have initiated a number of campaigns and recommendations aimed at reducing stigmatising media coverage (Mind 2000; Mindout for Mental Health 2005; RCP 2001; Media Bureau 2001; DOH 1999). Advocacy initiatives, developments in liaison, campaigning and health promotion are all playing a significant part in raising awareness and challenging negative attitudes. The media organisations themselves are responding with subtle changes in their portrayals including better informed reporting, more likeable and realistic characterisations and an increase in the utilisation of biographical style accounts. Some of these initiatives have led towards subtle yet important shifts in reporting styles such as the reduced association between mental illness and violence found by some researchers (Health Education Authority 1999; Francis *et al.* 2004). These developments all offer hope that a better representation of mental health issues can be achieved.

Definition of *positive*

The term *positive* might generally be regarded as relating to portrayals that challenge traditional stigmatising and stereotypical associations; those which educate and inform the receiver; and those which enable a sense of connection to be made with the person experiencing mental health problems. From a different perspective, *positive* might refer to a sense of personal or organisational gain. If we consider Berlo's (1960) communication model and the referent or stimulus for a particular message then the way in which *positive* is defined might perhaps be contested by different groups. Each group naturally will have their own needs and expectations that in turn impact upon the way in which messages are decoded and understood. The interpretation of media messages for example as being sensitive and supporting or patronising and unhelpful can be seen as being shaped by an individual's particular predisposition. Therefore, as with Jastrow's image (Figure 4.1), what we actually see, whether it be a duck or a rabbit, depends upon a range of influencing factors. How we see this image is governed in part by what we expect to see and what we want to see. Our orientation to a particular stimulus is fostered and influenced by our past experience and learning. We need also to consider the cues which are present, for example the labels or narrative content that help with comprehension. With the image in Figure 4.1, for instance, the title *rabbit* accompanied with a comment upon its long ears will help to focus the receiver's direction of engagement with it. It may at times, though, require extra coaxing to guide receivers away from particular readings of stimuli that are more familiar to them. From a mental health perspective, this can be seen in relation to the presentation of the message that the mentally ill do not pose a significant threat to the general public, a view that runs contrary to popular belief.

With regard to examples of positive mental health portrayal, it is worth clarifying what the term *positive* actually means as it may denote a number of different aspects dependent upon who is sending the message and who is receiving it. This is addressed in the following sections concerning the different groups of media provider, the mentally ill, and the mentally well. The terms mentally ill and mentally well are used here to provide a direct contrast with each other and the heading mentally well can be taken as referring to those who might perceive themselves to be free of mental health problems.

Media providers

We can look first at the media providers and what they might deem to be *positive* with regard to mental health portrayals. The most obvious factor here relates to the fact that 'madness' is an extremely attractive topic to media groups because of its selling potential. Commercial success will help to pacify and please the various stakeholders involved and perhaps ensure the continuation of a product. Mental health depictions are appealing and impactful and can have a major influence upon factors such as box office takings, television

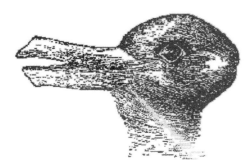

Figure 4.1 Duck/rabbit (Jastrow).

ratings, book sales, newspaper circulation and Internet site visitors. There are obvious pressures here to continue to use certain characterisations and terminology that have on past occasions proven successful. This is not to say that the use of overly dramatic or stereotypical representations is all bad as the high level of exposure achieved can play an important role in raising awareness if supported by opportunities for subsequent discussion and processing of issues. An example of this can be seen within the medium of television and the provision of information and contact details for self-help groups following the dramatisation of topics such as family abuse or self-harm.

The mentally ill

The issues of prime importance as regarded by those experiencing mental health problems concern those of accuracy, sensitivity and likeability. These messages are to be found within the media's vast output and have been stimulated by the growing recognition of the mental health service-user's voice and progress made through active campaigning, liaison with media groups and opportunities for direct expression through the media. The importance here is of providing the general public with a more realistic and accurate picture of the lived and felt experience of those with mental health problems. It also entails the portrayal of messages that are more normalising of mental illness as opposed to the generally depicted stereotypes of 'oddness', 'violence' or 'imbecility'. The importance here is of challenging age-old assumptions and associations and engaging the receiver with new and more productive ways of thinking. This helps to break down the 'us and them' barrier often found and fosters a greater feeling of connectedness. Magazine articles, television documentaries, autobiographical accounts and self-help Internet sites all include examples whereby the 'voice' of those experiencing mental health problems can be heard and whereby more informed and accurate role models are made accessible. Taking a slightly different approach, *positive* might also be regarded as relating to mental health media products that do not reflect negative connotations. Although not necessarily promoting positive associations either, the mere absence of a negative reinforcer can be seen as an improvement upon the generally found misleading portrayals. Although it is unlikely that sufficient numbers will exist for the process outlined by Skinner (1974) of extinction of the public's conditioned response to occur, it can certainly be perceived as a more welcome approach.

The mentally well

The term mentally well is used here to refer to those in the general population who deem themselves to be at the present time without mental health problems and is more of a perceptual opinion than anything based in fact. Two areas of importance for those in this category are education and entertainment. From an educative point of view, certain media products might be regarded as positive because of their potential to provide recipients with desired information. On the one hand, this might relate to an individual's need to learn more about the facts of mental illness because of genuine altruistic feelings. On the other hand, information might be sought as a means of coping with the anxiety and fear felt concerning the mentally ill or as a means of satisfying one's morbid curiosity about a fascinating and compelling topic. What is interesting, though, is the degree to which these recipients might accept various products as *positive* irrespective of the authority and accuracy of the information being provided. The other core strand includes media portrayals that are regarded as entertaining either because of their humorous or dramatic portrayals. These types of portrayal are certainly impactful and engaging and include some hugely popular examples such as the films *The Silence of the Lambs* and *Me, Myself and Irene*. While being applauded by many movie-goers as hugely entertaining and enjoyable they are at the same time rounded upon by mental health advocacy groups as being damaging and misrepresentative of those with mental health problems.

Altered thinking and creativity

When defining what is positive concerning the subject of mental illness it is important also to consider the degree to which altered states particularly within the domain of arts have been courted and even to some degree venerated. Whether it be through mental illness or chemical inducement, the changes in a person's thinking can be seen as helpful in providing direct access to untold expanses of creative thought normally unavailable to them. The sense of liberation created by altered thought processes and the productive drive provided by some mental health states are the main areas being focused upon here.

The evidence

A fair amount has been written about the links between mental illness and creativity although the evidence remains particularly uncertain. While there are a number of studies and reviews supporting a causal association between these two themes, they are not without their critics. Ludwig's (1995) study of 1,004 'eminent' people in creative professions found them to have higher rates of mental illness than those in the general population or eminent people in other walks of life. Another piece of research by Andreasen (1987) examined 30 creative writers finding a higher rate of mental illness than matched control subjects, a feature also true of the writers' first-degree relatives. Post (1994) investigated the backgrounds of 291 world famous men finding certain pathological personality characteristics and tendencies towards depression and alcoholism being causally linked to various types of creativity. These themes have also been studied in some depth by Jamison (1996) who demonstrated that mood disorders and artistic creativity tend to co-occur. The available evidence is fairly substantial although not without its detractors who view the research with concerns about methodology and lack of scientific evidence (Lauronen *et al.* 2004; Schlesinger 2002a; Waddell 1998). Another point of criticism is provided by Wright (1997) who contends that what the evidence mainly demonstrates is a more specific link between creativity and bipolar disorder and not the wider picture encompassing other mental health states. Schlesinger's (2002b) view is that the desire for a link between madness and creativity is in part generated through the idea that great talent coming from special suffering is romantic and thrilling. Despite the criticisms levelled at the available research, there are certainly grounds for considering the significance of this link: first, the wealth of historical and personal accounts that assert the importance that a person's altered states of thinking have upon the products being created; second, we might consider the desire of some within artistic spheres to actively seek altered states of cognition through psychotropic means in order to achieve a sense of creative expressiveness. Furthermore, we might also look at the significance that understanding the cognitive changes common to manic, depressive and creative states has in lessening the stigma of mental illness (Jamison 1989).

Jamison's (1993) study of living artists and writers revealed that most of them had high periods (mood changes) that were documented as coming on just prior to a productive period. This is supported elsewhere by theories that address dimensions of personality such as psychoticism, incorporating the two parts of thymotypy (working mainly through the mood) and schizotypy (working mainly through divergent thought). This, as Nettle (2001) states, facilitates the speed and range of imagination deemed so important for creative originality. It also provides the enormous energy required to drive on through a task in the absence of immediate rewards, especially in what are essentially solitary occupations and where critical feedback about a particular piece of work may be absent or only arrive years later. The periods of productivity following mood changes have been found in a number of creative and artistic people, for example Virginia Woolf who wrote that:

> one thing, in considering my state of mind now, seems to me beyond dispute; that I have at last, bored down into my oil well, and can't scribble fast enough to bring it all to the surface . . . I have never felt this rush and urgency before.
>
> (Woolf 1953: 74)

There are many instances where artists and writers have had access to divergent thought processes either as a consequence of their mental health state or as something induced through chemical means. It is perhaps the sense of disassociation and creative freedom that has been deliberately sought after by some, such as the writers Carlos Castenada and Aldous Huxley or the musician Syd Barrett. The feeling of cognitive liberation and creative expressiveness is a strong enticement and helps to explain why individuals such as William Blake are said to have actively embraced and even rejoiced in their madness. This is reflected by the degree to which Blake's madness allowed him to distance himself from the restrictions of worldly rationalism and embrace a new way of seeing the world around him. The notion being addressed here concerns the channels of expressiveness and lateral vision that are being opened up and are normally denied the majority. It reflects the views held by the avant-garde in Paris, of Flaubert, Baudelaire, Verlaine and Rimbaud, that true art sprang from the morbid and pathological. Furthermore it reflects the romantic notion that suffering and illness fired and liberated the spirit and that works of genius were in a sense hammered out on the '*anvil of pain*' (Nettle 2001). A number of classic works can be linked to this such as Malcolm Lowry's *Under the Volcano* or Sylvia Plath's *The Bell Jar* where these works of literature were in a sense directly fuelled by the authors' own personal experience of mental distress. A number of themes are related here including that of the creative genius suffering for their art. This is where great artists are drained and consumed by their talent, giving their all in the production of immense masterpieces. Certainly examples such as the composer Schumann and the legendary dancer Nijinsky fit this profile with their most productive periods being borne out of phases of mental illness and being in a sense eventually consumed by their art.

Just as the pyramids of Giza might be admired as a monumental achievement despite the extreme cost in human suffering, the admiration of great works of artistic or literary endeavour may take place in the absence of any real consideration for the toll exacted upon those behind them. It is a point reflected by Elizabeth Wurtzel in her book about depression, *Prozac Nation*. She writes:

> Forget about the scant hours in her brief life when Sylvia Plath was able to produce the works in Ariel. Forget about that tiny bit of time and just remember the days that spanned into years when she could not move, couldn't think straight, could only lie in a hospital bed, hoping for the relief that electro convulsive therapy would bring . . . think about living in depression from moment to moment, and know it is not worth any of the great art that comes as its by-product.
>
> (Wurtzel 1994: 260)

This is one facet relating to the concept that is mental illness but as expressed by Liz Sayce: 'It [Madness] is not irredeemably awful but mixed: at times tragic, wasteful, frustrating, boring, life denying; at other times extraordinary in the ways that contribute both to users' lives and to those around them' (Sayce 2000: 29).

Despite the various points addressed above, the association between madness and creativity is one that fascinates people and has not surprisingly proven an attractive lure to film-makers, something that is apparent in a number of recent films such as *Shine, A Beautiful Mind* and *Iris*. In these films we have a range of creative individuals whose talent provides the audience member with a strong point of contact overriding potential difficulties they might experience with that person's mental health state. Emotions are stirred within the receiver, such as feelings of sadness at the plight of John Nash (*A Beautiful Mind*) and Iris Murdoch (*Iris*) who are denied through their respective illnesses the talents that are most important to them. Likewise with the film *Shine*, the viewer is left with the uncertainty as to what extent David Helfgott's prodigious musical talent could have been developed further in the absence of his illness. What these types of portrayal importantly offer the receiver is a point of recognising the serious impact that mental illness can have on the lives of those affected. It takes the viewer to a position where they actually care about a person's experience and which generates a much greater sense of acceptance and awareness than might be otherwise achieved.

What's good about . . .?

As with the previous chapter, a variety of core media types have been selected with brief comments provided as to their positive potential with regards to the conveyance of mental health issues.

. . . Film

Connectedness

Film as a medium has the capacity to enable viewers to temporarily suspend their ordinary existence and to some degree become immersed in a new experience (Wedding and Boyd 1999). This experience sometimes involves entering the world of others and to a degree living and feeling experiences as if being directly involved. It might include gaining a sense of how altered states of cognition are perceived by the mentally ill but perhaps more importantly something of their felt experience. Some films, encourage a sense of connectedness and appreciation of a person's inner world, engaging the viewer with sensations such as hallucinations that are normally unseen. Polanski's *Repulsion*, for example, gives a very symbolic and observable representation of Catherine Deneuve's fragmenting world. Another example can be found with the film *A Beautiful Mind* where the viewer is presented with the same difficulty experienced by its principal character John Nash in spotting the distinction between reality and fantasy. The significance here is of the medium of film allowing what is normally unseen to be seen and what is unheard to be heard. Essentially, it enables the viewer to grasp something of what it might feel like to experience cognitive impairment and to subsequently foster more caring and nurturing feelings towards those concerned.

Caring treatment

Despite the number of films where treatment is depicted as a punitive or oppressive process there are some which show mental health care as a competent and caring process. These examples provide the viewer with a counter to the many negative stereotypes available and offer a sense of hope and reassurance in a system which individuals might approach with some trepidation. What is desired by many is the feeling that care is governed by the needs of the individual concerned and not by the system as is destructively shown in the film *One Flew over the Cuckoo's Nest*. Films such as *The Prince of Tides* and *Ordinary People* serve as positive advertisements for therapy by portraying an insightful and connected carer, someone who really does care. On a critical note, some of these films can be challenged for their lack of realism as they perhaps play into another stereotype with their dramatic and cathartic scenes. What does come across very strongly, though, is the message of recovery, that mental health problems can be overcome. This is aided in part by the concerned and caring helper or, as in the case of Dr Malcolm Sayer (as played by Robin Williams) in the film *Awakenings*, a tireless activist, prepared to risk all in the interests of their patients. What we get from films such as these is a sense of faith and optimism in mental health care that strongly contrasts against the showing of treatment as a destructive or punitive process.

Positive role models

The presentation of positive and likeable role models helps to counteract the usual association of unattractive and 'flawed' characterisations. The largely negative portrayal of the mentally ill as looking different or unattractive is similar to that of the disabled. Attractive or charismatic stars add a fresh appeal and foster a better climate for liking characters and in developing an enhanced sense of concern regarding their plight. Even fairly disagreeable or cantankerous characters such as Melvin Udall in *As Good As It Gets* come across in a favourable light. It is helped to some degree because we as an audience largely admire the actor Jack Nicholson and his character's warm side begins to emerge, enabling a more positive attraction to be formed. Other examples can be seen with the casting of Russell Crowe in *A Beautiful Mind* or Judy Dench in *Iris*, both attractive and popular stars. The importance for the viewer is in having aspects that help to develop feelings of attraction for mentally ill characters and subsequently help with acceptance of the 'whole' person.

... *Television*

Vicarious therapy

An important facet provided by the medium of television is its ability to help viewers feel supported and connected with others albeit vicariously. The television schedules are packed with shows that enable viewers to observe and learn from the problems encountered by participants or other viewers. Day-time television and the magazine-style formats offered by various stations include features about selected health matters, complete with phone-ins and 'your questions answered' by studio doctors such as Dr Hilary Jones. There are also a number of talk shows available to the viewer, some offering appalling examples of exploitation and participant abuse while others handle themes more sensitively and responsibly. To some degree, the latter type of example could be regarded as an on-air self-help group providing viewers who have experienced similar issues with a powerful sense of connectedness. This is usefully accompanied at the end of many such shows with contact details for related links and further information.

Education

The ability to inform an audience as well as entertain them about mental health issues is something that is strongly featured within the medium of television. This is achieved through a range of programme types such as news, documentaries, chat shows and features within breakfast and day-time TV shows. The public are offered different types of information depending upon the style of the show but these might include reports, case-study style information (as with documentaries), advice from health care professionals, or direct statements from television show participants about their experience of mental health problems. Television stations periodically place a strong focus upon education regarding mental health issues with short series of dedicated programmes, for example the BBC's *States of Mind* or Channel 4's *Inside My Head*. Short featured items with phone-ins and professional advice are regularly shown within the morning television schedules although these might be criticised for not adequately reflecting the full spectrum of mental health difficulties. The bias tends towards highlighting individuals whose plight is more sympathetically reviewed by the public as opposed, for instance, to the less comfortable subjects such as schizophrenia. An educatory function is also offered through programme types that, although being primarily geared towards drama and entertainment, carry enlightening mental health storylines.

Identification

Another regular means of engagement through the medium of television comes via what Horton and Wohl (1956) describe as parasocial relations and refers to a process of emotional identification whereby the audience relates to the experience of characters viewed on screen. This is found in particular with the prime-time dramas and soaps which regularly carry storylines with characters suffering from stress, emotional and psychological difficulties as well as relationship problems. Because many of these characters are so familiar to most of their audience, the feeling when watching them is that they are actually known to us. This is positive in that the sense of connectedness already felt with characters means that a greater understanding of and compassion for their distress can be achieved. The viewer can in a sense enter the world of the television character and to some degree connect with their experience, for example the emotional distress endured by Marlon in *Emmerdale* following the death of his wife or Sonia's emotional turmoil in *Eastenders* following the forced adoption of her baby. The significance, as illustrated by Livingstone (1998), is that viewers recognise and identify with the characters and experience them as real people, almost as if they were part of their family. It therefore puts us in touch with the lived experience and the feelings of those enduring mental health difficulties. These shows are on the whole extremely popular and achieve a large range of exposure.

. . . Literature

Inside looking out

Perhaps one of the most significant factors within the world of literature is the opportunity provided to enter the world of those experiencing mental health problems. This takes the reader into a position of connecting with a person's thoughts and feelings as opposed to the more familiar stance of observing them from a detached distance. This is achieved primarily through formats such as autobiographical writing or first-person narratives. To a certain degree we can regard autobiographical styles of writing as providing us with some of the most insightful and clear prose concerning issues of mental health. One might argue that it is the writing about mental illness by those who best understand the material being handled, having experienced aspects first-hand. These types of publication are currently highly popular and regularly feature as best sellers and include books such as Julie Gregory's *Sickened* (surviving Munchausen's syndrome by proxy) or Richard McCann's *Just a Boy* (learning to cope following his mother's murder by the Yorkshire Ripper). They also include publications that have won various awards, such as David Solomon's (2002) *The Noonday Demon: Anatomy of Depression* which was the Mind book of the year 2002. An extra feature provided by first-person narratives in fictional pieces of work is the ability to access places we would not normally be able to go, for example the emotional detachment experienced within the thoughts of the psychopathic killer (*American Psycho*) or the disordered and fragmented thinking within altered mental health states (*Briefing for a Descent into Hell*). These types of narrative provide the reader with a brief glimpse at the inner world of the person with mental health problems and consequently a greater appreciation and understanding.

Survival

In contrast to many media depictions where the person with mental health problems is either consumed by their condition or destructive towards others, is the sense of hope and optimism that comes through survival. These are found in abundance within both autobiographical and fictional types and provide a refreshing change to the often-found stigmatising alternative. The writing within autobiographical texts at times displays an immense degree of honesty and openness, as portrayed within Tony Adams' account of recovering from alcoholism (*Addicted*) or Paul Gascoigne's frank account of his personal problems (*Gazza: My Story*). This is also the case within a number of fictional accounts where featured individuals succeed in finding ways of coping with extreme life stressors that threaten to consume them (*White Oleander, I Know This Much is True*). Accounts focusing upon survival through adversity and hardship also focus upon collective experiences such as Mao's Cultural Revolution – two notable examples here being Jung Chan's *Wild Swans* and Hong Ying's *Daughter of the River*. These accounts are at times hard to read because of the extreme suffering being recounted although at the same time provide some very heartening images regarding the strength found to cope with extreme hardship and adversity.

. . . The press

Exposure

The degree of exposure offered through the newsprint media, aided by the high circulation some titles achieve, is an important factor with regard to positive health promotion. The significance of this is highlighted by the findings that newspapers provide us with most of our information about mental illness (Mason 2003). Although a fair degree of material accessed is neither positive nor accurate, there are a number of examples where care is taken to develop better and more productive messages. This is aided through various promotional campaigns as well as health information provided through featured articles, personal accounts, health advice and even to some degree the 'Agony Aunt' columns. The focus upon health promotion features very strongly within certain types of publication which include the better women's and men's magazines. There is a strong contrast found within newspaper types between tabloid and broadsheets as the former employs an overly stereotypical and sensational style of reporting whereas the latter features well within annual mental health awards for positive mental health coverage. Further exposure is gained when particular mental health issues are brought to the public's attention through the problems experienced by noted celebrities. Although not always sensitively handled, the better coverage provides others struggling with similar difficulties with feelings of connection and acceptance.

Liaison

The strongest liaison between media providers and mental health advocates has perhaps been developed within the newsprint media. The importance of increased involvement with those who better understand the nature and implications relating to mental health issues is reflected by various anti-stigmatising campaigns (*Changing Minds: Every Family in the Land; Mindout*; and *Shift*). Until recent years most liaison involved mental health professionals and the picture is now changing to encompass a variety of mental health service-user organisations. The significance of this is reflected in the Media Bureau's (2001) study *Mental Health and the Press* which found that only 6.5 per cent of all articles analysed included the voice of current or former mental health service-users. Many service-user organisations (e.g. Rethink, Mind, Zito Trust, Media Bureau) now actively prepare their members for getting involved with the media providing them with guidance, support and training days. Rethink in particular run a media volunteer scheme that puts journalists and broadcasters in touch with 'real experts' from a base of over 200 volunteers with direct experience of severe mental illness. These types of initiative help in directing journalistic personnel towards developing more sensitive and informed portrayals regarding mental illness.

. . . Internet

Accessibility

One of the most important qualities of the Internet is the ready availability of information on offer and the ease with which individuals can retrieve it. Recipients are presented with a vast storehouse of knowledge with material being posted from every conceivable viewpoint. This includes legislative material by the Department of Health, information about various conditions and treatments by health professional groups (e.g. the Royal College of Psychiatry) and supportive links by user–carer groups. This resource also offers immediacy with up-to-date material instantly available which is important concerning issues that need updating on a regular basis.

Empowerment

A core feature of the Internet is the opportunity afforded for those experiencing mental health problems in taking a more active role in their care. As individuals are able to seek out their own health information they are subsequently better informed and thereby come to health care professionals with a clearer understanding of their condition (Thede 1999). This has a number of implications upon the patient–practitioner relationship helping to foster shared decision making and the creation of a real partnership (Bauer 2002; Winker *et al.* 2000). It places a degree of power with the patient who is thereby better informed and more able to decide between available modes of treatment being offered.

Universality

The concept of *universality* can be understood as a process felt strongly by participants of group psychotherapy – feeling connected with others (Yalom 1995). The essence here is the sense of 'I'm not alone', as comfort and support can be obtained from the understanding that similar symptoms and difficulties are also being experienced by others. The Internet provides this facility both directly and indirectly. Direct support can be obtained through Internet support groups and various discussion room facilities whereby participants are provided with a vehicle for sharing and working through particular issues (Lamberg 2003). The feeling of connectedness can also be gained vicariously, by reading some of the many postings left by individuals and organisations concerning specific issues. This facility is particularly important for individuals who are experiencing difficulties in seeking help and may use this resource as an initial point of sharing or as a supplemental means of support (Oravec 2000).

Role models

An important contribution to the positive promotion of mental health issues is provided by the example of role models who share their distress and conflicts within a public arena and thereby remove some of the stigma attached. Such role models might mainly include well-known people although can also encompass non-celebrities who have a powerful experience to relate. Notable examples here include the revelations by Princess Diana about her problems with bulimia, of the Arsenal and England footballer Tony Adams concerning his addiction to drink, or even Kelly Holmes' account of her self-harming behaviour. Such examples as these reflect Bandura's (1986) social learning theory whereby learning can take place through observing another person modelling certain behaviours. It means that individuals who might be experiencing similar problems can gain heart from having a positive and powerful role model with whom to relate. In these instances, the public are provided with somebody expressing openly and honestly issues that are both deeply distressing as well as humiliating. What these examples significantly offer is a raised level of understanding and acceptance concerning the featured condition as well as a granting of permission to others to talk about and share their own experience. This is especially important with regard to topics that might otherwise be regarded as taboo, such as childhood abuse, so that many individuals do not deny themselves vital and much-needed support. The more certain aspects are shared, the more the climate is able to change to accommodate expression by others on related experiences. This can be seen in the steady increase in autobiographical accounts dealing with childhood trauma and abuse that now regularly feature on supermarket shelves and best-selling lists.

The way in which we respond to those in the public eye exhibiting mental health problems to a large degree relates to the affinity we already have for them. It is also interesting to note the sense of relish that may be exhibited by some concerning an individual's downfall, although it seems that this is mainly generated by the perspective from which their tale is told. If the individual concerned has direct access to the receiver then a more empathic and connected relationship can be achieved. The difficulty occurs when problems are related by an unconcerned third party (e.g. tabloid newspapers) with more interest in the 'scoop' obtained than the sensitivities of the person involved. The particular mental health state involved may also play a significant part with the more socially accepted forms of drug and alcohol abuse being treated more favourably than others such as schizophrenia. The type of coverage given by the media also plays a core role in helping the public appreciate and understand what a person's experience of distress actually entails. The largely detached and matter-of-fact reporting style reflected when, for example, stars book into a clinic for their next course of detoxification does not convey the desperation, isolation or humiliation endured by real people in real distress. It is mainly when the person is able to recount issues from their own perspective that public feeling becomes more sympathetic and understanding, which can again be illustrated by the case of Tony Adams who received a fair degree of media condemnation before finally being able to recount the story from his viewpoint.

The sense of acceptance provided by positive role models is also encompassed within the sense that mental health problems really can affect anyone. They are not conditions reserved solely for the obviously strange or more expected choice of individual but can literally affect anybody irrespective of their status. The famous role model, attractive, successful and adored provides a strong alternative to the classic stereotype of the mentally ill person and helps to challenge fixed views held by large sections of the public. This is aided through campaigns and initiatives engaged in by celebrities who help to promote positive associations of mental health. One example here is the collaboration between famous people who have endured mental health problems and health professionals to write what are essentially self-help books offering support and advice to others, for example Spike Milligan and

Anthony Clare's *Depression and How to Survive It* or John Cleese and Robin Skynner's *Families and How to Survive Them*. Other examples can be seen with their involvement in media initiatives such as the Headspace campaign, an exhibition by Mindout for Mental Health (2001b) where stars including Sting, Daniel Bedingfield, Romeo and Liberty X open up about personal difficulties they have suffered themselves or seen in others.

Positive role models provide those accessing media products with a much needed counter to the many negative role models whose destructive lifestyles have in some instances come to be admired or even venerated. This is especially true with regard to the destructive 'Rock and Roll' lifestyle that advocates a policy of living hard, and where dying young is a potential and accepted consequence. Many famous individuals within the music world have succumbed to this legend and the casualty list is littered with high profile stars such as Jim Morrison, Brian Jones, Janis Joplin and Jimi Hendrix. These are chaotic and tormented individuals who have tragically been consumed by their difficulties as an adoring yet fairly unconcerned public watches on. In more recent years the Nirvana singer Kurt Cobain successfully committed suicide after a number of failed attempts. Another tortured musician was the Manic Street Preachers' guitarist Ritchie Edwards who disappeared a number of years ago. He had a history of self-harming behaviour and would even cut his arms on stage accompanied by the cheers of fans. This in a sense illustrated something of the rock and roll myth, the legend that self-destructive and hard living behaviours are to some degree expected or even demanded by their fans. What are needed instead are role models who illustrate and portray something different, expressing the true nature of problems without glamorising them and advocating support-seeking instead of self-destruction as the way forward. This is why, for example, Tony Adams stands as a much more vital and productive role model than, for instance, the footballer George Best.

Service-user expression

In recent years there have been numerous developments and initiatives aimed at promoting the artistic expression of those affected by mental health problems. This importantly recognises the right and need of anyone affected by mental health difficulties to have access to various channels through which to communicate their experience. It also provides others with valuable opportunities to gain greater awareness and insight into the thoughts and feelings concerning a person's felt experience of psychological distress. It is in a sense the learning about mental health issues from those who best understand them (Rogers *et al.* 1993). Another core feature here is the fact that creative expression is encouraged and accessible, in principle, to anyone affected by mental health problems and not something that is reserved solely for the artistic genius. This is matched by the public's growing acceptance of and interest in the personal reflections of 'ordinary people' as reflected in the huge popularity of autobiographical narratives that are steadily attracting both critical as well as commercial acclaim. One of the most significant factors concerning a person's involvement with creative or artistic expression is the potential therapeutic value that is gained. This is highlighted by a number of authors who state that the very act of writing has proven beneficial in helping them to work through and resolve personal issues (Pegler 2003; Lott 1997). Writing has an extremely powerful therapeutic potential as illustrated by McArdle and Byrt's (2001) study that employed the medium of literature with mental health service-users and reported some positive treatment outcomes. It is also worth noting that there are now some specific publishers such as Chipmunkapublishing that cater specifically for individuals who are survivors of mental health problems and wish to promote better attitudes towards mental illness.

There are a number of national and local initiatives and projects that have encouraged and even celebrated service-user expressions. One initiative of particular significance has been the Royal College of Psychiatrists' (2001b) *A Mind Odyssey*, launched in 2001 to help inspire both mental health care professionals and service-users in expressing their creativity through various forms of the arts (RCP 2005). This has led on to the creation of a range of locally organised exhibitions including the 'A Mind Odyssey: Diversity' programme of events offered across the city of Leeds in October 2003. The sheer diversity of expressive types is illustrated through the wide range of activities covered including the forms of art, photography, dance, drama, writing, music, poetry and film. These events were organised and led by a variety of individuals from the voluntary sector and the National Health Service and involved people who have used or worked in mental health services.

The encouragement and development of service-user modes of expressions are importantly helping to normalise the experience of mental illness with the message that anybody can experience psychological distress. The provision of direct access to a person's thoughts and feelings means that what has traditionally proven a frightening and to some degree avoided topic can now be better addressed and understood. Historically, the societal approach was to distance and rid itself of madness by segregating and removing those designated as being so afflicted. The present climate of community care and high media exposure means that different approaches are needed including better education and to some degree a process of desensitisation. Service-user expression offers countless benefits to both those experiencing mental health problems as well as others who are better able to connect with and understand them. It also helps to reduce some of the stigma involved by creating a more open and accepting climate in which people are more able to talk about and share experiences without the fear of being rejected, ridiculed or alienated.

Promoting mental health

When looking at the dynamics and processes involved with mental health promotion certain core features stand out. Changing people's attitudes towards a more accommodating and understanding approach requires a certain degree of education. This is vital if individuals are to be helped to make better sense of the messages they are exposed to including the ability to discriminate between positive and stigmatising material. As well as addressing a person's requirement for accurate information is the need to tackle the emotional aspects (e.g. fear and anxiety) that keep people with mental health problems segregated and at a distance. This means developing greater feelings of connectedness with not only the person but also the topic of mental illness. One of the main problems facing those involved in health promotion is how to most effectively produce and disseminate their material to make it as widely accessible as possible. This involves getting their material noticed, certainly something that is important given the wealth of stimuli they have to compete against. Therefore two major issues which health promotion needs to address are those of education and exposure.

Education

A prime factor in helping to shift misconceptions and inaccuracies regarding mental health issues is the exposure to reliable sources of information and messages that inform people about what is actually occurring. This is recognised by various campaigns and strategies such as the Royal College of Psychiatrists' Changing Minds: Every Family in the Land campaign or the Mindout for Mental Health's (2001a) *Mindshift: A Guide to Open-minded Media Coverage of Mental Health* which both, among their various targets, seek to promote a better understanding of the real nature of mental illness. Among the various anti-stigmatisation approaches being employed are projects specifically geared towards better education. One such scheme is the Mental Health Awareness in Action programme of educational workshops set up in West Kent schools to help tackle stigma and discrimination (Pinfold 2003). The main aims of the workshops were the promotion of the messages that:

- We all have mental health
- Mental health problems are common
- Mental health problems are different to learning difficulties
- People can recover from mental health problems
- The discrimination that people with mental health problems feel is damaging and hurtful
- Any link between mental health problems and violent behaviour is a myth

The emphasis of these workshops was on discussion and engagement with these issues as opposed to a simple reception of imparted information. Prior to the workshops most information that participants had received regarding mental health issues were cited as being primarily from the various media sources or their parents. There was a significant change in attitude noted as a result of this programme in that the language used to describe the mentally ill replaced derogatory phrases and stigmatising terms with more sensitive and accepting words. This scheme in particular illustrated the fact that raising awareness and improving understanding about mental illness helps to facilitate and accommodate better attitudes being developed towards mental illness. The success of workshop-like events such as this is illustrated by Haghighat (2001) as being largely due to the opportunity for individuals to ventilate their anxieties and feelings. This is an important point and worth noting as informing people about the low risk in reality posed by those with mental health problems may on its own be insufficient. Many people need the opportunity to express and understand what their fears are actually based upon if they are to be able to accommodate and consider this point properly.

The liaison between mental health advocates and media groups is another core approach that is helping to tackle misrepresentations and promote more accurate messages. It involves media groups working directly with mental health professionals and those who have experienced psychological distress. These links have steadily developed with both service-user organisations and mental health professional groups providing training and support for their members who wish to get involved. These initiatives have on the whole been widely welcomed although in some instances are viewed with concern. In particular, Persaud (2000) reflects upon the involvement of service-users and questions how in touch some of the media's favourite pressure group leaders might be with medical research and practice. He also criticises the fact that they are in some instances called upon for comment before medical practitioners with considerable experience. This argument perhaps plays down the very real importance of allowing the public to be addressed directly by those who it might be argued have real expertise to speak upon topics concerning mental illness. The point in question here concerns who is regarded as having the most authority and expertise to speak about a mental health condition – those with years of professional experience or those with years of personal experience. The main issue, however, is to achieve the right balance with both health care professionals and service-users being employed by various providers of media services. Persaud (2000) raises an interesting question concerning the ways in which spokespersons among service-users are selected. It is, though, an aspect that relates equally to health care professionals. Obviously media personnel will have their own favourites, a choice that is assisted by accessibility or the particular mental health topic being addressed. While mental health advocates are steadily developing their liaison role, Cuenca (2002) feels that health care professionals need to recognise the power of the media and to increase their involvement from that of isolated individuals to that of a collective group. The continued development of these relationships should help to foster more positive and less distorted messages about mental illness and mental health professionals. This relationship also involves to a certain degree of educating and challenging the attitudes held by those within the media because, as Salter (2000) points out, informing the public is not necessarily the journalistic profession's primary motive. Clearly, financial considerations and the dramatic and impactful potential provided by the topic of mental illness will also feature strongly.

As well as educating the public about aspects of mental health the media also provides a function for educating health care professionals. This is illustrated by Wall and Rossen (2004) who highlight the potential for developing critical thinking skills through using the media as a teaching strategy. This is done by enhancing students' sensitivity to the personal experiences of mental health service-users and broadening their understanding of mental illness and its treatment.

Exposure

One of the greatest difficulties facing those involved in mental health promotion concerns the issue as to how to make their message stand out and get it noticed. Certain media channels and products gain high exposure rates and would be ideal vehicles for positive health messages but they may prove prohibitive in terms of access. Austin and Husted (1998) reviewed the experience of developing media programmes through several broadcast and print formats and found a number of restrictions in terms of cost effectiveness and space available to carry messages. New media products such as the Internet provide wonderful opportunities for making wide ranges of material easily accessible and are commercially viable options to develop. It is a means that enables material to be disseminated and available to people instantly across the world, although this obviously relies upon those searching the Internet being able to find the site.

The issue of exposure relates to the number of people who have access to messages being sent out. In terms of developing awareness and understanding of mental health issues, the initial input could be of a positive or negative type, the importance being a person's noticing of the material and the opportunity to challenge and reflect upon it. This means that even products such as television soaps that rely upon dramatic and stereotypical imagery can be potentially beneficial if this leads to an eventual raising of awareness. Another useful example is provided by Lars von Trier's film *The Idiots* which could be regarded as offensive and insulting or alternatively can be viewed as challenging and thought provoking, depending upon how it is understood. This film focuses upon a group of people who deliberately present themselves as being mentally handicapped in order to evoke a reaction from the public and who purposely use stereotypical presentations including the word 'spass' as a means of provocation and confrontation. It is a powerful film that challenges the audience members to consider their own discriminatory attitudes and potential feelings of discomfort relating to behaviours that are 'strange' and 'embarrassing'. This relates to a major theme involved within health promotion, that of social exclusion, and the extent to which we might play a part in its perpetuation. The exposure provided by blatantly negative exposure could also be productive if followed up by immediate protest or comment as seen, for example, by *The Sun*'s U-turn following the complaints received regarding their initial appalling coverage of the news that Frank Bruno had been involuntarily admitted to hospital for depression. The importance here is the exposure that more productive messages can subsequently achieve as well as the opportunity for the public to be informed that what it was initially in receipt of was actually incorrect.

A degree of exposure is necessary in order to help positive imagery stand out and be noticed amidst the vast array of negative and stereotypical messages. As illustrated by Broadbent's (1958) filter theory, the amount of information passing along the input channels (sensory system) is far too much and would overload the brain with too much information to assimilate. A filter is followed by a bottleneck (limited capacity channel) that selects some of the incoming messages for processing by the brain to regulate the intake (Figure 4.2). There is a short-term storage facility for input not initially selected, although these impulses become weaker with time if not accessed.

What is important here is the extent to which particular messages stand out as obviously some will attract more attention than others and increase their likelihood of passing into the brain for processing. A difficulty facing those engaged in health promotion concerns the simple fact that positive images on the whole are far less appealing and impactful than their negative and dramatic counterparts. The high degree of impact evoked through the sensationalist reporting of a high profile news event such as the Soham

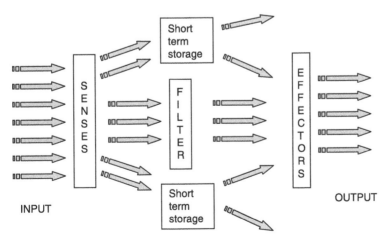

Figure 4.2 Adapted Broadbent's filter theory (1958).

murders is hard to match for sheer emotional intensity. The steady diet of negative reporting along with the periodically dramatic 'Psycho Killer' type of headlines is unnerving and unsettling. It is subsequently hard to put ones fears and uncertainties to the side even when confronted with information to the contrary. The messages mostly portrayed within the media would seem to suggest that those with mental health problems are on the whole unpredictable, potentially violent, unsuccessful, asocial or eccentrically odd. The fact that some individuals fit this profile does not equate with the erroneous assumption that all of those with mental health problems must do so as well. The problem here is of regarding the mentally ill as a unified 'mass' instead of a collection of unique individuals with their own individual sets of experiences. In some cases it is only when people get to hear first-hand of an individual's experience of psychological trauma that their attitudes about mental health issues start to shift. It is perhaps still a very slow process with those 'telling their story' being separated out from the 'mass' rather than any real reorganisation of attitudes and beliefs taking place. This is because of the pervasive and insidious power that the steady drip of negative imagery and messages has upon our values and beliefs. It might be interesting to view the public's relationship with mental health issues via the following equation:

1 High profile media story $= x$ (media campaigns + positive storylines)

The value for x is the aspect needing to be determined although it can generally be regarded as being greater than 1. This all means that health promotional campaigns have to create products which are able to compete against and challenge messages that on the whole have a greater intensity and emotional resonance. The way forward is obviously a combination of approaches working at both challenging and questioning negative media messages while at the same time promoting more realistic and productive alternatives. It means helping to educate people but at the same time tackling the fears and anxieties that restrict any real attitudinal change. Getting messages noticed through dramatic means is proving useful, something for example portrayed within television soaps that are first engaging their audiences through entertainment and dramatic means and then taking the opportunity to present new associations and educative messages. Even though some of these are still far from perfect because of the unrealistically rapid shifts between illness and wellness the overall degree of exposure and ability for viewers to engage *with* the mentally ill character is a positive achievement. This coupled with helplines and contact information helps to make the coverage of mental health themes more favourable. This forms in part the essence of positive mental health promotion, which involves: normalising mental health topics and encouraging people to talk about them; presenting more of the person's lived and felt experience thereby making their actions and behaviours more understandable and consequently less frightening; educating people as to what is fact and what is fiction. These types of approach will help to reduce some of the distance felt between those with mental health problems and those who deem themselves to be mentally well thereby reducing some of the painful and alienating consequences of social isolation.

5 The news media

Introduction

This chapter focuses upon the medium of news reporting and the way in which mental health issues are reflected in newspapers and magazines. The emphasis is placed here upon the printed news medium as other formats such as those provided by television and the Internet will be addressed in subsequent chapters. The significance and importance of news information is illustrated by the view that television and newspapers come ahead of family and friends or other sources of information when it comes to influencing opinion about mental illness (Mason 2003). While television news is seen as being characteristically thin in content (McNair 2003), exposure to information in newspapers enables a lasting impression on memory to be obtained (Robinson and Levy 1986). The printed news medium therefore offers scope for greater depth of coverage as well as acting as a reinforcing agent for stimuli accessed through other sources.

It is interesting to consider the issue as to how we learn about the world around us as well as the range of sources accessed from which we derive our news. In the current era of multimedia, *news* is accessed whenever we pick up a newspaper or magazine, turn on the TV or radio or log on to the Internet. This process is added to by what we learn through social interaction from others who have been exposed to these sources. The *Oxford English Dictionary* defines *news* as 'newly received information about recent events or matters of topical, local, or personal interest' (OED 2005). It is through this process of inputting incoming stimuli that our understanding and learning about the world around us is obtained. These stimuli carry messages which may be regarded as single information chunks or collectively as news. The printed news media is accessed in conjunction with other media formats and may involve minimal amounts of time compared to our use of television, the radio or the Internet. A study into how we engage with different media types found the 'average' person in Britain spends about 20 minutes per day reading a paper as opposed to 3.8 hours watching TV and 3 hours listening to the radio (Kent 1994). This obviously raises the question as to which media type is the most influential with regard to developing attitudes concerning the topic of mental illness.

One of the first issues related to accessing the news concerns that of choice and deciding upon which information sources to select from. Almost 200 years after the invention of printing, the first recognisable form of newspapers became distinguishable from the pamphlets and newsletters of the sixteenth and seventeenth centuries (McQuail 2000). Since then the range of publication types has developed into an almost limitless array of titles to choose from. In the case of newspapers, choice is offered initially by national and local press and then by broadsheet and tabloid style presentations. The presentation of news in the printed format is widened further with the large availability of women's and men's magazines, specialist interest publications and professional journals. Readers are drawn towards particular titles by virtue of their attractiveness, informational value and appeal. Choice is influenced by a range of issues such as the style of presentation used, the political or social stance reflected, accessibility and the degree of influence exerted towards certain titles by peers and family members. While most readers retain a regular choice of newspaper or magazine, some are periodically swayed by the coverage of big news stories and the captivating titles and images displayed prominently on the front pages of other publications.

The way in which news items are packaged is influenced by the needs and expectations of a publication's target market. A clear contrast can be found between broadsheets that carry a more detailed and sober style of reporting and the more simplistic and moralistic tabloid style. The largest selling types of magazine available are women's magazines with different interest groups and ages being catered for by separate publication types. While the predominant focus appears to be upon glamour and fashion, other main themes include lifestyle issues such as cookery and comfort-living, 'people' stories and health matters. There are also the 'coffee-table' type publications that attract their readers with promises of the latest celebrity stories and dramatic features of coping with trauma and hardship. There are also a growing number of magazines aimed at a teen and pre-teen market that use attractive and popular television and music stars as their main selling point. A further strand of news is obtained from specialist titles with most interest groups being represented within the spheres of leisure and sport, social issues (e.g. *The Big Issue*) or professional groups.

The above publication types provide the reader with a vast range of presentation styles with their various means of attracting attention and meeting the requirements of their readership. For example, a clear contrast can be noted between the dramatic, sensational and easily accessible tabloid style and the more contemplative and less subjective broadsheet approach. What we learn in terms of news can be regarded as being heavily dependent upon the source accessed and the manner in which information is relayed. This information will vary widely as regards degrees of accuracy and detail of reporting. This all raises particular concerns around whether or not the more reliable items of news can be extracted from the overall mass as well as the degree to which it is interpreted and understood correctly.

The current picture

There have been numerous reports highlighting the fact that coverage of mental health issues within the press is predominantly of a negative nature with many age-old stereotypes being reinforced (Health Education Authority 1999; Mind 2000; Mindout 2001; Day and Page 1986). A study of 1,999 newspapers in terms of mental health coverage revealed dangerousness to be the most common aspect covered and it was rare to find stories of accomplishment or recovery (Wahl 2003). Calls for the reporting of mental health issues to be improved have been made by many parties and indeed a study carried out by the Media Bureau (2001), *Mental Health and the Press*, found that many journalists themselves (64 per cent) believed that coverage should be better.

One of the main problems resulting from negative coverage is the effect upon those experiencing and living with mental health problems. The Mind (2000) *Counting the Cost* report surveyed 515 people with mental health problems living in England. Over half of these said that negative media depictions made their mental health problems worse. A third said they felt more anxious and depressed as a result of bad press and one in twelve said that they felt suicidal as a consequence. The key messages emerging from this report highlighted that press coverage is poorly balanced, reinforces stigmatising portrayals, has a negative effect on individuals' mental health and perpetuates social exclusion. The sensationalising of news items does not demonstrate adequate sensitivity or responsibility to many concerned, a point strongly illustrated by Richard McCann in his book *Just a Boy* about his struggle to cope with the newspaper coverage of his mother's murder by the Yorkshire Ripper.

What comes across strongly from these studies and reports is the overwhelmingly negative coverage of mental health issues reflected through news stories. It is especially disconcerting when considering that this source generates most of our learning about mental illness (Mason 2003). A bit of comfort perhaps can be derived from the subtle shift demonstrated in recent years with a small increase in positive imagery and educative messages being shown (Health Education Authority 1999). The broadsheet newspapers and certain women's and men's magazines in particular have devoted space to articles and features relating to the active promotion of mental health matters.

Regulation and guidelines

With regard to the world of publishing, the issue of ownership is a significant factor as owners have a major influence upon the presentation of news stories and features (Hetherington 1985). From a mental health perspective, therefore, it is discouraging to note McNair's (2003) assertion that the ownership of the British national press continues to be concentrated in the hands of a few publishing organisations. Unlike other news sources such as 'new media' and the Internet, the overall degree of impartiality or freedom within the print media is restrictive with fewer perspectives being represented. At times, it is questionable as to whose interests are best being served by particular news stories. While writers might maintain that the interests of their readers are being served, there are clearly also commercial considerations that have to be addressed in order for a publication type to remain operational. This raises the issue as to what control or checks are in place to maintain a sense of balance between the interests of these two parties. On occasion, when reading headlines which 'scream out' such terms as 'Mad Psycho' or '*Silence of the Lambs* Maniac Freed to Kill', one might be forgiven for assuming that newsprint was a totally unregulated media where subjective opinion was the accepted norm. The reality is that journalists work within what is mainly a self-regulating industry and have various sets of guidelines that advise against these styles of reporting.

The first Royal Commission on the press introduced voluntary self-regulation in the form of the Press Council in 1947. This was established in part as a response to public and parliamentary criticism of declining press standards (Calcutt 1990). It was not particularly successful and the failure of the Press Council seemed to be related to the fact that it had no formal code of practice as to what the press should and should not be doing, nor any legal powers of enforcement (McNair 2003). The main thrust of the Calcutt Committee's report (1990) was for continuing self-regulation by the press and the replacement in 1991 of the Press Council by the Press Complaints Commission (Snoddy 1993). As Petley (1999) indicates, the PCC is regarded as being largely ineffective as we only need to immerse ourselves in the daily, debased reality of a large amount of the British press to understand why the PCC cannot be taken too seriously as a regulatory body.

Previous versions of the *Code of Practice* of the PCC have been replaced with the newly revised (2005) code which has added a few extra clauses and altered the wording from *should* to *must* in an attempt to strengthen their members' compliance. Selected clauses from the PCC indicate the huge gulf that exists between the ideal and the reality of press reporting as illustrated by Clause 1 (*Accuracy*) and Clause 12 (*Discrimination*).

Clause 1 – Accuracy
(i) The Press must take care not to publish inaccurate, misleading or distorted information, including pictures.
(ii) A significant inaccuracy, misleading statement or distortion, once recognised must be corrected, promptly and with due prominence, and where appropriate an apology published.
(iii) The Press, while free to be partisan, must distinguish clearly between comment, conjecture and fact.
(iv) A publication must report fairly and accurately the outcome of an action for defamation to which it has been a party, unless an agreed settlement states otherwise, or an agreed statement is published.

If we consider the impact that certain types of presentation may have, one might argue that the damage is not so easily undone. An apology may seem fairly insignificant when compared with the destructive nature of stereotypical terminology or imagery often used. An aspect pointed out by those experiencing mental health problems is that of feeling stigmatised and alienated by the predominantly disparaging reporting styles used. This has a marked impact upon individuals' self-esteem and confidence, significantly affecting numerous aspects of their lives. It is questionable, therefore, as to how much the damage is redressed by the offering of an apology.

One of the issues here depends upon the perspective from which we are viewing material. Although potentially offending a number of readers, from an editor's point of view, subjective, emotive and stereotypical language may be seen as justified. A headline such as 'MAD PSYCHO KILLER ON THE LOOSE' emerges forcibly from the page and demands immediate attention. Such a presentation leaves the reader with a sense of unease that may be fully out of context with the actual threat posed. For a start, headlines are in larger font and placed in a predominant eye-catching position on the front of the newspaper. Any resultant apologies may be placed somewhere inside the newspaper in small font, in a place which is very easy to miss or ignore. What is needed perhaps is to create a similar impact with a newspaper having to give up their headlines to: 'NEWSPAPER PRINTS INSENSITIVE AND MISLEADING MENTAL HEALTH STORY'. This ideally would then be followed up with a new, balanced and sensitive article promoting a more accurate and positive mental health view. As it stands, particularly in the case of tabloid reporting, this is unlikely to change much as commercial considerations continue to strongly influence and dictate styles of reporting.

Clause 12 – Discrimination
(i)   The Press must avoid prejudicial or pejorative reference to an individual's race, colour, religion, sex or sexual orientation or to any physical or mental illness or disability.
(ii) Details of an individual's race, colour, religion, sexual orientation, physical or mental illness or disability must be avoided unless genuinely relevant to the story.

This clause appears to be frequently ignored with the continuation of stereotypical and stigmatising notions such as the association between the concepts of *mad* and *violent*. The term mental illness is also, as Philo (1996a) and Wahl (1995) indicate, used as a metaphor to represent features that include helplessness, violence or mental handicap.

A regulatory aspect, although perhaps loosely linked, is libel law which protects a person's right to reputation against defamatory allegations. This was defined by Lord Atkin in 1936 as: 'Any publication which tends to lower the plaintiff in the estimation of right-thinking members of the public generally' (Petley 1999). However, this raises the question as to what opinion 'right-minded' people hold about the theme of mental illness, especially in light of Bloch and Singh's (1997) assertion that it represents one of the most stigmatised conditions worldwide. Therefore, the frequent discriminatory and unrealistic portrayals offered by the press seem to match the overall picture found in society. A core issue then concerns the opportunities that those in this group have of representing themselves and of speaking out against defamatory and misleading statements. Traditionally the mentally ill were regarded as a group of individuals who did not have a collective voice or sufficiently strong advocates who were willing to act on their behalf. Fortunately this picture is starting to change with many instances of editors and writers being challenged, about stories they have written, by professional and voluntary organisations such as Leeds Media Minders, a group of service-users and mental health workers who actively encourage liaison with and feedback to media providers.

Other guidelines have been developed within the journalistic industry to guide its members such as the National Union of Journalists' *Code of Conduct* (NUJ 1999). Clause 3 of this code states that: 'A Journalist shall strive to ensure that the information he/she disseminates is fair and accurate, avoid the expression of comment and conjecture as established fact and falsification by distortion, selection or misrepresentation' (NUJ 1999). This reflects the sentiments as expressed by the PCC with terms here such as 'accuracy', 'falsification' and 'misrepresentation' standing out. We can again challenge these points particularly considering the regular distortion and misrepresentation that takes place within the print media. One highly misleading issue in particular relates to the widely held view that the mentally ill pose a significant risk of violence to the general community. As a number of studies indicate, there is no significant risk posed by this group and they are far more likely to harm themselves than they are to harm others (DOH 1999). The public's general unease about mental illness is firmly highlighted by the fact that they are more at risk from young men under the influence of alcohol (DOH 2001) or those using recreational drugs (Repper *et al.* 1997) than they are from those experiencing mental health difficulties. Another significant issue relates to the question as to what accuracy actually means. There are many ways in which misconceptions may be fuelled by an insensitive choice of subjective and slang terminology. Consider, for instance, *The Sun*'s 'Bonkers Bruno . . .' headline regarding the boxer Frank Bruno's hospitalisation for depression. This understandably was met with a severe backlash from the general public and a number of mental health organisations. No direct apology was given for their coverage of a story that appears to contravene Clauses 1 and 12 of the PCC *Code of Practice* (2005). *The Sun* newspaper did, however, respond quickly with a subsequent edition of their paper carrying the headline 'Sad Bruno in Mental Home' and a day later initiating their fund for mental health charities. While the newspaper can be commended for acting swiftly upon this matter, the second headline seems hardly an improvement and their mental health fund might be viewed from a cynical point of view to be geared more towards protecting their readership than in addressing the feelings of Frank Bruno or others who might be affected.

One aspect influencing poor reporting of mental health issues is concerned with a writer's lack of understanding or experience regarding the reality of mental illness. In an attempt to address this, various guides aimed specifically at journalists have been produced. An example of this is the *Guide for Journalists and Broadcasters Reporting on Schizophrenia* (NUJ/RCP 1999). This has been developed in collaboration between the NUJ and other bodies such as the Royal College of Psychiatrists and Schizophrenia Ireland. It is an informative and well-presented guide challenging some of the widely held misconceptions such as the association between schizophrenia and split personality as well as the much-misrepresented connection between mental illness and violence. Another example is the booklet *Severe Mental Illness Explained – A Guide for Journalists* (DOH/Rethink 1999). This guide was developed by Rethink (a leading mental health charity) in collaboration with the Department of Health. This guide similarly explores and challenges some of the stereotypical and stigmatising attitudes towards mental illness and provides factual information regarding schizophrenia and personality disorder as well as challenging violence myths and concludes with the section 'Reporting without Stigma'. These types of guides are extremely valuable and highlight the developing collaboration between media providers and mental health advocates.

Liaison

When looking at a number of poorly constructed or overly dramatic stories we might be forgiven for thinking that nobody of any experience or reliability has been consulted and that the story's sensationalism has been preferred over that of accuracy. This is despite the steady increase in involvement between media personnel and professional organisations or service-user groups. While the longer-established links are with health care professionals there is a growing voice among those who have experienced first-hand mental health problems. Besides complaining and offering feedback about negative media coverage, service-users are becoming more active in liaising with media providers and involving themselves more directly with broadcasting and publication initiatives. This challenges the historical trend of the mentally ill being treated as if they have little of credibility or value to offer. It means that journalists are encouraged to look beyond the tried and trusted health care professionals, the people who might be generally regarded as being able to supply more reliable information. As Potter (1998) highlights, most are chosen on appearance of their expertise and their willingness to tell a good story. Official sources, such as professional organisations, are often preferred as journalists and editors believe that they have important things to say and accept the information provided as factual, thereby eliminating the need to double and triple check facts (Paletz and Entman 1981). Reliability is obviously a core factor but it also points towards a lack of trust in the voice of experience by the mentally ill.

A study by the Media Bureau (2001) *Mental Health and the Press* found only 6.5 per cent of all articles analysed include the voice of current or former mental health service-users (either individual or group). Most journalists said that the main barrier to contacting people with mental health problems was that they were not sure who to contact or didn't include their perspective because a number of individuals didn't want to be named or photographed. There are two core issues here, that of preparing news personnel to access service-users and that of preparing service-users to involve themselves with media groups. First, we might consider the pro-activeness or the accessibility of service-user groups in coming forward and making contact with news agencies. It also involves training and preparation for members and their involvement. The Media Bureau's (2001) study found that the biggest barrier for service-user groups getting involved with local or national newspapers was in not knowing who to contact and a fear of negative coverage. Only half of the individuals who made contact had their views published although most were pleased with the results and the accuracy shown by journalists. This applied more so to the national than to the local or regional press. This involvement will hopefully develop further and has been made a priority by a variety of service-user organisations such as Rethink, Mind, the Zito Trust and the Media Bureau who actively prepare their members for working with media providers by offering guidance, support, workshops and training days. This reflects the strong moves being made by professional groups such as the Royal College of Psychiatrists and British Psychological Association that recognise the importance of preparing their members for a greater involvement with the media.

The best and the worst of news reporting

The type of message being transmitted through the print media will evoke a corresponding reaction in its readers. With regard to mental health content, this may fall somewhere on the *connecting–distancing* continuum reflecting perhaps the largely polarised portrayals of mental illness, either depicted as a survivable condition or as a destructive force. The latter view is clearly the predominant depiction, that of mental illness as a negative, deteriorating or destructive condition. The opposite pole from this presents a more hopeful aspect where we may be heartened by astonishing tales of courage and survival or simply provided with accurate facts about mental health issues. It is not always clear as to which type of message is being transmitted as there may be a confusing plethora of ambiguous sub-texts and images, all of which serve at the same time to educate and mislead their readers.

Mental illness as a destructive force

The core theme here relates to the destructive nature of mental illness either to the individuals themselves by self-harm and neglect or to others through violence and intimidation. Although various studies actually highlight the fact that those with mental health problems are significantly at risk themselves from the public or actually pose a greater risk to themselves than to others (DOH 1999), the predominantly reported association is of the mentally ill representing a threat to other people (Philo *et al.* 1996). This is reinforced by the findings of Nairn *et al.* (2001), with mental illness depictions being predominantly negative and consistently linked with the characteristics of violence, failure and unpredictability.

These are very strongly held views with a sense of threat and unpredictability being attached to the mentally ill irrespective of the nature of their actual condition. This point is highlighted by Wahl who asserts that:

> It is not simply that the image of people with mental illness as violent and criminal appears so often and in so many different sources that troubles mental health advocates, it is that this image is characteristic of media portrayals ... When one sees or reads about a person with a mental illness in the media, it is more likely that the person will be shown as criminal or dangerous than in any other way.
>
> (Wahl 1995: 65)

An interesting example of this can be illustrated by the *Daily Mail*'s article concerning the murder of a young American artist in a London park and their headlines 'Four Hundred Care in the Community Patients Live near the Murder Park.' In the middle of a lengthy report was a brief statement by the officer in charge of the case stating 'there was no evidence yet that Muller was attacked by a person with mental health problems and that police were keeping an open mind on the motive' (Main 2003).

Some of the responsibility for the media amplification and public panic, according to Morrall (2000b), rests with the psychiatric disciplines for not acknowledging the gravity of the problem and failing to offer the public appropriate reassurance. This is an important point as in a sense the public need to be debriefed and helped to place high profile murders in context. The typical media scrimmage that followed the conviction of Ian Huntley over the Soham murders appeared to highlight the public's perceived desire for every scrap of information possible. This is a familiar process that has been seen in other devastating high profile events such as the Hungerford massacre or the Dunblane tragedy. Clearly, public attitudes are influenced and hardened towards the mentally ill following such traumatic public events and Appleby and Wessely (1988) noted following the Hungerford massacre a significant increase in agreement with the statement 'people who commit horrific crimes are likely to be mentally ill'. It also assists in placing the mentally ill into a separate category from 'normal' murderers, being construed as double trouble, *mad* and *bad* (Morrall 2000a).

There are a number of negative consequences presented by unbalanced media reporting that focus strongly upon the risks that individuals with mental health problems pose to themselves and others. The publicity connected with these has contributed to an unbalanced policy debate and measures introduced in response to public fears have served to impose additional constraints on people with mental health problems (Hallam 2002). Aided by such coverage, the public and politicians are led to believe that unless people with mental disorders are segregated from the general public the streets will not be safe. This misassumption is aptly summed up by Taylor and Gunn's (1999) analogy that the odds of being killed by a mentally ill person are the same as those of winning the National Lottery.

There is certainly a wealth of evidence to suggest that the effect of reading newspaper articles reporting violent crimes committed by those with mental health problems has a particularly destructive influence upon people's attitudes (Mason 2003). Howlett (1998), however, provides a contrasting view, analysing data from a 1997 MORI national survey of attitudes towards mentally disordered offenders and mental health services. He argues that media focus on homicide and violence by mentally disordered offenders does not increase stigmatisation and that, on the whole, both positive and negative imagery are presented within the media. While there is some support for this argument it perhaps fails to recognise the impact that may be created by a single negative storyline that has a more pervasive and impactful effect than a number of other educative and health promotional messages.

There is a need to maintain the subtle modifications in reporting styles which have been noted over recent years. Wahl, Wood and Richards (2002) examined changes in newspaper articles between the years of 1989 and 1999 and although noting that dangerousness was still the most commonly reported theme in 1999, the incidence portrayed was less than that of a decade earlier. It is also helped by first-person accounts addressing the reality of living with a mental illness. The journalist Ingrid O'Gunleye writes in *The Independent on Sunday*: 'It does not help that most people have the wrong idea about a psychotic person, often accompanied with screaming tabloid headlines. I am only a danger to myself and not to other people' (2003: 1). It is an extremely open and frank account that in a sense stresses the sensitivity that needs to be demonstrated by those responsible for carelessly portraying mental illness. Poor reporting styles serve to add to the sense of alienation and persecution felt which in turn influence negative outcomes such as self-harming behaviour.

While destructiveness displayed by the mentally ill towards others is greeted with fear and trepidation, when it is turned inwards the reaction is generally very different. The reporting here may be largely absent unless detailing the plight of a noted celebrity. Witnessing the downfall of famous individuals appears in some cases as a type of *schadenfreude* (joy at the misfortune of others), something that is almost gleefully celebrated by the media and the public, especially when linked to a sex scandal. In other cases, where individuals are universally liked, the reaction may be geared more towards emotions such as sorrow and pity. This is exacerbated by the use of words or phrases that evoke sympathy such as the term 'sad', as featured in the headlines concerning the plight of Frank Bruno 'So Sad' (*Daily Mirror*) or Kerry McFadden's hospitalisation for depression towards the end of 2004 'Sad Kerry in Clinic' (*The Sun*). While an improvement upon other styles of reporting, the tendency in some cases leans towards reporting styles that employ past-tense phrases and regard the person as 'pathetic'.

A further issue concerns the over-selling of glamour and the unattainable goal of perfection sold prolifically through large sections of the media. The disturbing nature of associated learning is reflected in a number of studies that focus upon body image perceptions following exposure to various magazines. Martinez-Gonzalez *et al.*'s (2003) study reported disturbing findings of a higher risk of incidents of eating disorder from those having a high exposure to girls' magazines. This reflects the findings by Hamilton and Waller (1993) which showed that acute exposure to media images can increase body dissatisfaction in anorexics and bulimics. Similarly, studies by Cash *et al.* (1983), Stice and Shaw (1994) and Durkin (2002) revealed that participants exposed to idealised female images in magazines demonstrated a reduction in body satisfaction and an increase in levels of depression, shame, insecurity and guilt. The unrealistic sense of self is also promoted within men's magazines with the creation of the fantasy of modern men who can work long hours, develop new and satisfying relationships with women and children while preserving their bodies against ageing and decay (Jackson *et al.* 2001). These types of portrayal foster the same kind of problems found with women's and teen magazines with unrealistic and unattainable goals being offered up and a subsequent infusing of anxiety and critical self-approval with regard to one's own presentation. The steady diet of enticing, glamorous and largely unattainable messages has an insidious and detrimental effect upon many individuals' self-perception. As illustrated by Wykes and Gunter this is largely caused through the internalisation of socio-cultural messages reflecting that: 'The ideal self-image may be considered as either an "internal ideal" or a "societal ideal" resulting from the dictates of the surrounding cultural and societal environment as to what constitutes the perfect body' (Wykes and Gunter 2005: 4).

Mental illness as a survivable condition

A significant contrast to the recognition of mental illness as a destructive entity can be found in a number of publications presenting a positive alternative. This is where mental health problems are seen as being survivable and where a more sensitive and realistic portrayal is demonstrated. These types of depiction highlight the fact that anyone might succumb to the pressures and stresses of life and experience mental health problems. They include detailed and informative articles, inspirational and heart-warming tales of survival, frank and honest accounts of problems experienced as well as features and advice concerning health issues. These types of presentation encourage better responses towards the subject of mental illness by encouraging feelings of connectedness with another person's lived experience and by offering a contrasting point of view to the wealth of misleading messages encountered elsewhere.

Within the newsprint media, *survival* stories are largely found within magazines and feature both celebrities as well as unknown members of the public. They include examples such as:

- The comedian Hugh Laurie's account of his experience of depression and how he overcame it with the aid of psychotherapy (*Woman*, 15 July 2002).
- The Irish actor Colin Farrell recounting how he was assisted by his psychiatrist to cope with his drug problem (*Best*, 16 December 2003).
- TV chat show host Trisha's history of personal and family mental health problems and related problems of panic attacks and depression (*Now*, 12 March 2003).

Survival stories can be heartening and it is encouraging to note the extent to which people are able to cope with extensive amounts of trauma, heartache and distress and yet still appear to have a reserve of strength and optimism with which to face the future. For some readers this will provide them with role models they can identify with and from whom they gain some inspiration towards discovering and developing their own means of coping. These features are usually brief and contain a 'happy ending', written at a point when individuals are beginning to overcome their difficulties, have come to a sense of resolution and are subsequently able to rebuild their lives. The celebrity articles in particular are important in reducing some of the stigma associated with mental illness. A number of campaigners hope that the increasing willingness of stars to talk about their mental health problems will help lift the taboo surrounding mental illness which is a strong aim of Mindout for Mental Health's (2001b) Headspace campaign. The difficulty faced here concerns the polarisation of attitudes, noted by some mental health charities, concerning different types of mental illness, notably with young people hardening in their views towards patients with schizophrenia or serious mental illness yet sympathising with those who are depressed or distressed (Rethink 2004).

Dramatic, emotive and stereotypical reporting stirs up the public's passions and helps with sales. The same can be true of positive mental health reporting but perhaps with a very different set of feelings being evoked. In place of fear, outrage and concern we have those of pity, sympathy and hope. While negative coverage has an all-pervasive distancing quality that marginalizes and segregates those experiencing mental health problems, positive coverage can be defined primarily by material that increases understanding and acceptance. It enables the reader to engage in a brief feeling of connection with the individual involved either through sympathy for their plight or through being heartened by their struggle and survival. These types of article can be received in a different light although it needs to be recognised that for a number of individuals the pitying and sympathetic coverage will be felt as patronising and disempowering.

Magazines present us with a variety of information types, with fashion, feature articles and health issues perhaps predominating. This is borne out by a content review of teen magazines which found fashion topics to be the dominant subject (35 per cent), followed by an emphasis on feature articles (interpersonal relations), self-esteem issues, special problems, beauty, entertainment and special recurring columns that offer tips and advice (Evans *et al.* 1991). There is some room for optimism with regard to the coverage of mental health issues in popular periodicals which over recent years have demonstrated both an increase in articles featured as well as changes in terminology with less stigmatising terms being used (Wahl and Kaye 1992). This is a welcome aspect especially when coupled with the high exposure attained by some publication types such as women's magazines with circulation rates that can be measured in millions (Borman 2003). Certain regular features such as health sections, featured articles and even agony aunt columns provide the reader with optimistic and supportive messages relating to mental health issues.

A number of magazines carry regular features and pages offering health advice which is listed under headings such as 'Mind, body and soul' (*Prima*) or 'Beauty and health' (*Elle*). These include information such as 'Stressbusters', *Marie Claire's* top ten techniques for tackling stress. They are usually presented in a very reader-friendly format with language very much geared towards their targeted audience, for example 'Sorting out the Mr rights from Mr wrongs can take its toll on your time and energy . . .' Other versions include the case-study article, questionnaire-type format and 'agony aunt' advice column. The 'agony aunt' column has undergone a fair degree of change over the years with some now offering much more constructive and supportive advice including links to self-help groups and organisations. For example, while *New* magazine's Jane O'Gorman's advice is fairly general in nature she importantly offers a variety of links to specialised agencies, such as women's aid helplines, self-harm organisations, Cruse and Relate, for further contact and support. This reflects Winship's (1987) assertion that the modern day 'agony aunts' support rather than blame women, encouraging them to be self-assertive about their needs. The total range of advice offered covers the spectrum from insensitive and careless through to the supportive and helpful. Another issue for the reader to consider concerns the qualifications of the person giving advice as in some cases few credentials are indicated. Where recognised professional qualifications are provided the reader is offered a measure of reassurance, for example *Prima*'s Dr Sarah Brewer who is listed as a GP and specialist in complementary medicine and herbal medicines.

There are a number of positive presentations found within feature articles, for example *New Woman* magazine's (May 2004) focus upon three women with mental illness that carries the introductory comment: 'They're young, attractive and successful. But Liz, Emma and Sharon all share the same problem. They all suffer from a mental illness' (*New Woman* May 2004). Another example from *Prima* (May 2004) helps reduce some of the stigma attached to mental health problems by showing three 'ordinary women living normal lives'. What these types of representation do is to reflect either attractive and successful role models or those that are simply 'normal', a far cry from the often-employed unattractive and unsuccessful stereotypes. Features such as this go a long way to normalising mental health problems as well as challenging the myth that once diagnosed one can never completely recover. The essence being portrayed is not necessarily that of complete cure but one of learning to accept and cope with particular difficulties. It is perhaps a more powerful message than the illness–wellness polarisation and brings us into a closer proximity with mental illness and an understanding that psychological distress can co-exist with coping and wellness, and that the mentally well can experience mental health difficulties and that the mentally ill can experience wellness.

News framing

Clearly, the format or packaging of news is geared towards the perceived needs of the audience. As Murdock states:

> Having selected an event for presentation as news, newsmen face the problem of placing it within a context that will render it meaningful to the majority of their audience. Necessarily therefore news presentations must work with meanings and imagery which are both widely available and generally understood.
>
> (Murdock 1998: 208)

This perhaps explains the narrow language base used by the tabloid press or the clear similarities in presentation found between various titles.

Another factor concerns the positioning of news articles within a publication where a sense of imbalance may be apparent. The Glasgow Media Group's study of press content found that negative mental health images tended to receive headline treatment while positive items were largely 'back page' in their profile (Philo 1996c, 1999). As Kress and Leeuwen (1998) highlight, newspaper front pages provide different degrees of salience and framing to material and thereby endow them with particular values. This can distort the actual newsworthiness or significance of particular stories as their importance is reflected in the number of column inches taken up, the font size employed or their placing within a paper. We can already reflect that:

> Of the millions of events which occur every day in the world, only a tiny proportion ever become visible as 'potential news stories'; and of this proportion only a small fraction are actually produced as the day's news in the news media.
>
> (Hall 1981: 234)

Therefore, the irresponsible front-page coverage that alarms the reader with the sensationalised association between mental illness and violence places the whole issue out of its real context. With mental health issues, the difficulty for many readers lies with their lack of experience and knowledge and their subsequent difficulty in discriminating between what is factual and what is not. With regard to front-page coverage, there are a number of instances where featured items are clearly not the most important or newsworthy item, as can be illustrated by the extreme focus within the tabloid press upon David Beckham's broken metatarsal prior to the 2002 World Cup.

A further issue relates to that of noticeability and which stories in particular stand out from the wealth of news items being covered. From a perceptual point of view the most apparent item might be that which is placed forcibly before our consciousness by virtue of its front-page treatment or through the inclusion of striking images or of emotive language. As many people's reading habits might be fleeting and passive, reporters and editors find attention-grabbing techniques very appealing. This poses a difficulty for those concerned with mental health promotion which is unlikely to gain the same impact as that of a tabloid style headline such as 'Cannibal Psycho Killer on the Loose'. People are drawn towards the dramatic, the scary and the sensational, all of which tend to perpetuate their continued use by the press. It is certainly evident that normalised stories concerning mental illness are almost invisible by contrast.

Informing or misinforming?

The reporting of news can be regarded either as a reflection of what is occurring in society or as a construction by journalists. News, according to Potter is: 'a creation resulting from the active selecting and interweaving of images into a processed reality. . . . they [journalists] are strongly influenced by elements outside the event, such as their deadlines, space limitations, and their own news sense' (Potter 1998 : 111).

The process of news construction includes aspects such as selecting what gets covered, deciding upon what will become the focus of the story (or the hook to interest people), as well as determining how the story is to be told. In some cases this involves manipulating reality, which according to Shoemaker and Reese (1996) involves the media emphasising certain behaviours or including stereotypes. It can further be illustrated with the inclusion of factual inaccuracies, such as that observed by Crepaz-Keay (1996) that over the 18 months of the Boyd inquiry into homicides and suicides by discharged mentally ill patients, the actual reported frequency of such deaths was doubled by nearly all newspapers. There have been a number of calls for greater responsibility to be shown in reporting with even 64 per cent of reporters themselves noting that it should be better (Media Bureau 2001). Allan (1999) echoes this with the statement that journalism should be committed to truth and upholding the various codes of newsworthiness. There is an issue here, though, concerning what exactly the term *truth* means and whose *truth* is being told. Hall *et al.* (1978) argue that news organisations do not merely report events but are active agents in constructing the socio-political environment that frames those events. Journalists therefore contribute significantly to the process of where and how problems are defined. Other writers indicate a deviancy amplification model whereby public indignation or moral panic concerning a type of 'deviancy' may be fanned (McNair 2003). Much of this is heavily influenced by commercial considerations with publishers very mindful of what generates the largest audience with the presentation of deviance proving attractive and newsworthy (Potter 1998). The bottom line for many, therefore, is the fact that no newspaper can achieve adequate sales and survive unless it has a clear concept of what will interest its readers. A paper is packaged or presented in ways that will attract attention and hold its audience (Hetherington 1985), a factor that picks up Kalbfleisch's (1979) three basic ingredients for a 'top story' of insanity, unpredictability and victimisation of ordinary people. Indeed, the pressures to get the best story are aptly reflected by Belsey who states: 'The doctor who exploits a vulnerable patient for sexual favours can be struck off . . . an accountant who steals from a client can be sent to prison, but a journalist who misbehaves may get a scoop and a promotion' (Belsey 1998: 5).

Reading the news

A person's understanding of news items is influenced significantly by the way in which material is packaged and formatted. We can regard the style of news presentation being subject to a range of considerations not least the type of publication and audience expectations. For example we can look at titles such as *The Times, The Sun, Hello* magazine, *Cosmopolitan* and *The Big Issue*, as having a diversely different readership and consequently varied formats. Clearly, each publication type will have a view as to the distinct needs and desires of their readers, an important consideration linked to subsequent sales. In order to briefly reflect upon these differences, the comparison of publication types will centre around three different titles, *The Times* (broadsheet), *The Sun* (tabloid) and *Now* (popular magazine) with regard to their coverage of Frank Bruno's involuntary hospitalisation for depression in September 2003. The main focus is upon the tabloid and broadsheet style with the magazine example being included as a further point of interest. These articles will be reflected upon in relation to the messages conveyed through headlines, images and narrative.

Headlines

On the whole tabloids favour eye catching, jargonistic or humorous headlines, whereas broadsheets opt for a more objective and informative style. The tabloid approach is one of quickly engaging the reader, rousing their curiosity to want to learn more of the dramatic and engrossing tale promised by the headline. The headlines are often enriched with adjectives usually associated with mental health problems and some of the references made seem almost incidental, in a number of cases having little relevance to the story being recounted (Vousden 1989). Emotive or dramatic words stand out and the intention is clearly one of attracting readers who might be perusing the various titles on offer. In sharp contrast, the broadsheets present succinct terms that serve to a greater degree to alert the readers concerning some of the information to follow.

When considering the range of headlines depicting news of Frank Bruno's distressing condition, the most obviously damaging and insensitive headlines were provided by *The Sun* with their first edition headline 'Bonkers Bruno Locked Up'. This naturally resulted in a fierce outcry and condemnation from many parties and a statement by the mental health charity SANE read:

> It is both an insult to Mr Bruno and damaging to the many thousands of people who endure mental illness to label him as 'bonkers' or a 'nutter' and having to be put in a mental home ... we call upon newspapers involved to apologise to Mr Bruno and to all those who experience the stigma such attitudes inflame.
>
> (SANE 2003)

A fair degree of criticism centred upon the paper's headline which was roundly condemned for its insensitivity and poor choice of words. The paper's initial concession was a rapid change of headline within later editions of the paper to the perhaps equally bad 'Sad Bruno in Mental Home'. Along with the paper's subsequent launching of a mental health fund were printed comments that alluded to the interest and concern that they have afforded Frank Bruno throughout his career (*The Sun* comment, 24 September 2003). From a cynical point of view this appears to be a blatant attempt at bolstering the paper's image in light of its badly calculated choice of words. Tucked away within this piece is the line '*To us he's one of the family*'. It comes across almost as a desperate attempt at reassuring their readers that the paper, like millions of their readers, really does care about.Frank Bruno after all.

A quick glance at other tabloid headlines illustrates the fact that a lack of sensitivity and stigmatising language was also being displayed by others in this newspaper type:

- 'Bruno Put in Mental Home' (*Daily Express*)
- 'So Sad' (*Daily Mirror*)
- 'Sick Bruno in Siege Drama' (*Daily Star*)

These headlines provoke misleading interpretations and serve to reinforce a number of classic stereotypes with words such as 'Mental Home' (associations such as *mentally defect or learning disability*), 'Siege' (*drama, crisis and danger*) and 'Sad' (*an object of pity or someone pathetic*). Some of these terms reflect Bagnall's (1993) reference to the language used within the tabloid press as *popspeak*, having a strong ritual flavour and using a small stock of recognisable words.

Interestingly, although using very different language, the broadsheets appear to have their own small collection of words and phrases to choose from. This is illustrated by the following:

- ' "Depressed" Bruno sectioned under Mental Health Act' (*The Times*)
- 'Depressed Frank Bruno is sectioned under Mental Health Act' (*Independent*)
- 'Frank Bruno Admitted for Psychiatric Treatment at Hospital' (*Guardian*)
- 'Frank Bruno is Sectioned under Mental Health Act' (*Telegraph*)

These headlines collectively inform the reader as to the essence of the story – that of Frank Bruno being involuntarily committed for mental health care owing to depression. Further information is provided by *The Times*' use of inverted commas around the term depression implying that his diagnosable mental health state has not yet been publicly confirmed.

Surprisingly though one of the most positive headlines was provided by *Now* magazine with 'Frank's Biggest Battle Yet'. This headline is both positive and optimistic, alluding to the fact that mental health problems can be overcome. He is also affectionately referred to by his first name only, reinforcing the personhood of the individual within this story and reflecting something of the degree of affection with which he is held by a large majority of the population. This seems to be more in tune with *The Sun*'s claim of 'To us he's one of the family'. When addressing the impact upon the general public we have the contrast between, on the one hand, messages that tend to work by provoking an emotional reaction and, on the other, those that are objective and informative. As tabloid newspapers reach a much wider readership we can infer that many stereotypical associations will be perpetuated and accepted by a largely unquestioning audience.

Images

The stories and narrative accounts being conveyed within the print media are complemented by the inclusion of pictures that further develop the overall set of messages that are to be sent out. The perceptual receipt of these images can be understood though a semiotic approach whereby aspects within a visual array have particular meaning for the observer (Harris and Lester 2002). The publication types under discussion used some very different types of imagery, each leading the reader towards a particular set of messages or associations. *The Sun* for example chose to include as its most prominent picture a photograph of Frank Bruno in pantomime costume holding the glove puppet Sooty. This, in relation to the story being conveyed is at best a poorly chosen one and at worst an attempt to see him because of his mental health problems as an object of ridicule or derision. It does not in any way convey the true seriousness of mental illness and only serves to reduce his credibility further. Other images featured by *The Sun* show his wife Laura looking stressed and upset, an ambulance leaving his home, a boxing ring he had installed in his garden and a final picture of Frank the World Boxing Council (WBC) champion. Some of these images seem almost randomly selected or chosen to specifically highlight his eccentricity, as with the case of the boxing ring and pantomime shots. The ambulance is shown for no real purpose other than the dramatic nature of Bruno being taken away from his home. This seemingly random assortment of images has been carefully selected reflecting some of the qualities of visual stimuli identified by Berlyne (1960), that elicit attention from their recipients: intensity, contrast, change, movement, novelty and incongruity.

In contrast to this, *The Times* chose a single picture on their front page, that of Frank holding aloft the WBC belt after having triumphed in his fight against Oliver McCall in September 1995. This depicts Frank simply as the popular hero, in sharp contrast to *The Sun*'s depiction of clown. *The Times* followed this up in the next day's paper with a collection of shots far more sensitively chosen than those appearing in *The Sun*. The first two featured his wife Laura looking worried and drawn and Frank with his hand to his head as if in exasperation. This was followed by a collection of eight images, all of them, apart from one (victorious in the ring and disbelieving), of a smiling Frank. It is in a sense a greatest-hits montage of photos charting his personal and professional triumphs. These pictures tell their own story and highlight the great affection held by the public for Frank the *person*.

The personal view also featured very strongly in *Now* magazine where he is pictured in a suit after a night out. This is not Frank the public persona (boxing hero or clown), but simply Frank the person doing ordinary things. The picture is accompanied by the caption 'Frank looked drawn on a recent night out in London'. It is a well-chosen image, which evokes feelings of sympathy for the person that is Frank Bruno.

Narrative

Some of the fundamental differences between broadsheet and tabloid news-papers may be reflected in the view that broadsheet readers seek new ideas to make them sit up and think whereas popular paper readers want stories that fit their current conception of the world and not one that will disturb it. As Allan (1999) states, British tabloids provide varying degrees of depth regard-ing straight news although each places a premium upon entertaining as opposed to informing the reader. The preferred modes of address are straight talking, snappy headlines and everyday vernacular to enhance popular appeal. Pursehouse's (1991) analysis of interviews with British tabloid readers indi-cated that the tabloids are regarded as offering respite or distraction from tasks that require concentration. They were not seen necessarily as a reliable source of balanced reporting with most readers looking towards the medium of television for their 'real news'.

A number of these issues are reflected in *The Sun*'s article which says very little about the nature of mental illness other than reinforcing a number of stereotypes. In particular, phrases are included from unclear sources includ-ing how he at times slept in a boxing ring or tent in his garden as well as the statement, 'At the weekend it was claimed that he had started believing he was racing legend Frankie Dettori'. No information is given as to who it was claimed by and it seems only to have been included because it fits the classic popular behaviour patterns of the mentally ill. The notion of source is an interesting one, and *The Sun* primarily seeks boxing personnel for comment. The only medical source is a retired neuropathologist asked for comment to help make the weak link between brain damage caused by boxing and Frank's mental health state. No real information about the true nature of mental illness is given and it amazingly takes the boxing promoter Frank Warren to provide any thoughts as to diagnosis.

All of this seems contrary to the National Union of Journalists *Code of Conduct* (1999) Clause 3 with regards to accuracy. *The Sun*, along with other tabloid titles has rightly in this instance met with broad condemnation over their handling of this story and a number of statements were released by mental health charity and advocacy groups over the handling of this story: 'The shameful tabloid media treatment of Frank Bruno is unfortunately reflected in the day to day experience of 630,000 people with a severe mental illness who are too often shunned by society' (Cliff Prior, Chief Executive of Rethink 2003). Richard Brook, the Chief Executive of Mind, issued an open letter to the Editor of *The Sun* newspaper stating:

Despite recent improvements . . . your news reporting has historically been an area of grave concern and has often caused a flood of complaints into Mind. *The Sun*'s reporters have been short-listed or awarded Mind's Bigot of the Year Award more times than any other national newspaper. Only a long-term overall editorial commitment will address this. Failure to do so will suggest that the paper's actions on Monday evening, to change the headline, were forced by embarrassment rather than representative of journalistic integrity.

(Brook 2003)

This last point is certainly one worth addressing. The backlash from readers and mental health advocacy groups will have certainly caused some discomfort prompting them, a day later, to launch their own campaign for mental health titled '*The Sun*'s Fund for Bruno'. This fund was promoted with emotive terms such as 'Dig deep . . . like Bruno did for Britain' and cynically perhaps kicked off with a £10,000 donation. This response might reflect what Eric Berne (1964) refers to as *good games*, that of being helpful to others but with an ulterior motive. In this instance the change of moralistic stance from 'Bonkers Bruno' to staunch mental health advocate is certainly helped by protecting their commercial interests.

In contrast to the tabloid style, the broadsheet coverage has been less sensational and more concerned with presenting the facts in a more concise and objective style. Unlike the tabloid presentation, this story was not the main feature in any of the broadsheet newspapers and in the case of 'The *Guardian* did not even make the front page. *The Times* article uses words sparingly and avoids using the titillating details included by other papers. It is a more sober piece of reporting which informs the readers succinctly as to the nature of 'sectioning', Frank's boxing career, family problems and something of the wide-ranging affection felt for him by others. Bias in the tabloids is blatant and unashamed, bombarding the reader with emotive words and phrases whereas bias in the broadsheets may consist of omission of certain facts or selected quotes (Bagnall 1993). The broadsheet language used is kinder, such as the phrase 'Two uniformed officers . . . spent four hours persuading Bruno to go for treatment', whereas the same detail was reported in *Now* magazine as 'police took three hours to remove him'. The *Now* magazine style incorporates elements of the tabloid style with a number of stereotypical details, such as Frank believing he was Frankie Dettori and a comment from a nightclub owner stating that, 'we knew as soon as he spoke that he'd lost it'. These are unnecessary details other than to dismiss the experience of those experiencing mental health problems. This article, though, does include a significant comment from the mental health charity Mind that appears a welcome inclusion and in part challenges some of the stigmatising messages addressed elsewhere in this article.

In sharp contrast to the quality broadsheets that are widely regarded as being more informative, the reporting style in the popular press focuses more upon emotive and sensational content omitting a fair degree of contextual evidence (Chalaby 1998). The style of presentation employed reflects the informational requirements of their targeted readership as people obviously differ in their generalised motivations for learning and their willingness to confront new messages. As Slattery *et al.* (2001) indicate, the broadsheets are aimed at those at the higher end; the active seekers who are interested in all kinds of information whereas the lower end is geared towards those exhibiting a low level of interest in accessing new learning. To some degree, the issue affecting those at the lower motivational end can be reflected in Chalaby's (1998) view that they may not be aware that they are particularly missing anything and consequently do not feel the desire to seek out added information. The concern here relates to the fact that most of the information actually accessed contains a large degree of inaccurate and misleading content. As with the perceptual image in Chapter 2 (Figure 2.3) of the *old woman/ young woman*, unless alerted to the presence of another way of interpreting this picture the observer may not feel the need to search further, retaining solely their initial perception.

Engaging with news

With regard to news accounts, at the heart of the process of inclusion and exclusion are 'frames' or 'principles of organisation' which work to impose order on the multiple happenings of the social world so as to render them into a series of meaningful events (Goffman 1974). Critiques of news coverage include the metaphor of a mirror being held up to reflect the social world and the amount to which distortions have been allowed to creep into the reporting process, coupled with vast numbers of 'blind spots' (Allan 1999). This clearly highlights the importance relating to the writer's background and the particular version of events we are subsequently exposed to. It might be illustrated on a large scale by the circulation of propaganda messages within, for example, the communist bloc regimes and the deliberate extent to which the public might be misinformed of events occurring in the wider world. A subtler example could be seen in the reporter's lack of knowledge about mental health issues and the inclusion of inaccuracies within their writing. Readers might take for granted that what they read in their chosen newspaper or magazine has a good degree of accuracy because of the strict regulatory structures that are available to govern what is written. Information and advice are received generally in good faith with few opportunities to stop and challenge it or to find out how credible the writer's base of experience is. Readers might be particularly interested to note the extent, or even lack of research, consultation and personal experience that have played a part in informing the writer as to the facts being reported. The negative association with mental health issues is heavily reflected in styles of reporting across all newsprint formats and includes broadsheet as well as tabloid reporting. One study in particular focused upon the print media in three countries (UK, USA and Australia) and reviewed 118 articles over a one-year period, accessing two broadsheets from each country. The predominant tone relating to mental health issues in all three countries was negative, more so in the UK (Priebe 2003). The tabloid format, however, contains more stigmatising messages than their broadsheet counterparts (Peters 2002). This is also borne out by

Mind's (2000) *Counting the Cost* report with regard to the best and worst coverage of mental health issues within different publication types where respondents saw the best coverage being employed by the broadsheets and the worst by the tabloids.

Our concept of news or what is regarded as *reality* can be seen as being created through the social process of communication sent out by the mass media (Johnson-Cartee 2005; Nimmo and Combs 1983). The stream of messages received are filtered through an individual's own perceptual screen and developed further through discussion with others. The chain of communication from sender to receiver is fraught with difficulties influencing the overall fidelity of this process. Some journalists and writers refute notions of subjectivity in their accounts and support the 'mirror on society' approach by arguing that a number of journalists in a room together will all produce the same story (Chibnall 1981). McNair (1998), however, argues that many journalists fail to recognise that in their selection of facts and in their contextualising of them, they are creating news by giving such facts 'meaning and context' when they are transformed into a story or narrative. It is also perhaps hard to ignore the fact that many will also have an eye on how the final product will be received and engaged with by their targeted audience. This helps to explain the divergence in reporting styles whereby journalists writing for different publication types address their readers with an appropriate level of linguistic complexity and sophistication (McNair 1998) as well as degrees of emotive and dramatic engagement. Although being influenced significantly by the sender, the reader brings their own personal interpretive diversity from which to decode facts. As McQuail (1997) states, this depends to a large degree upon the social position and outlook of the receiver who subsequently fits the facts accessed into personal frames of interpretation and relevance. This process is supported by Potter (2004) who outlines the process of filtering that is applied to the process of reading whereby individuals screen out material that is deemed as irrelevant for their purposes. The primary need, though, is for media providers to change in their reporting styles towards a more sensitive and responsible style of coverage. There are some indications that this is starting to shift, as outlined earlier, with a number of initiatives being employed. These include campaigning, liaison with media providers, health promotion schemes and educative messages. Progress is minimal, although there are small signs of change as indicated by the Health Education Authority (1999) as well as Mind's (2001) inclusion of fewer articles in their annual shortlist for bigot of the year.

Conclusion

The overall picture with regards to news reporting of mental health issues suggests a slight positive shift over recent years in what remains though a largely negative style of coverage. Various initiatives have aided in the promotion of better mental health coverage such as the developing collaboration and liaison between news personnel and mental health advocates. This has resulted, in some instances, in a better-informed and more thoughtful style of reporting. It is concerning however, that the strides taken with regards to the positive coverage of mental health issues found within the broadsheet press is not reflected by what is produced by their tabloid counterparts. As the tabloid press have a much higher sales circulation it could be assumed that the majority of readers are still exposed to regular messages that report upon mental health issues in a sensationalist and emotive style, with a common usage of stereotypical representations. A problem facing those involved with the promotion of mental health concerns the attractiveness of certain styles of coverage both to press personnel and their readers. It takes a case such as *The Sun's* temporary transformation to mental health campaigner (following complaints received about their coverage of the Frank Bruno story) to suggest that the overall picture can change. The main factor here however related to the fact that this was a much liked and widely respected figure. There is also the issue regarding the type of mental health problem reported to consider as a diagnosis perhaps of schizophrenia would not arouse the same degree of sympathy and concern. It seems that a major change in societal attitudes is still needed before sufficient pressure is brought to bear upon those producing the news.

6 Literature

The medium of literature

The medium of literature offers something uniquely different to other media sources such as television or film. While these other types of media communicate through the combined modes of narrative, imagery and sound, literature provides us with messages primarily through the narrative format. It is in a sense left to the reader to construct their own perceived images and understanding from the text laid out before them. The writer acts as a guide, evoking feelings and creating meaning through the richness of their narrative. It is a medium that has limitless potential, constrained only by the limitations of the writer's craft or the reader's imagination. The literary genre has the potential for a deeper level of engagement with characters than that offered by other media formats. This is achieved through the ability to take the reader directly into a person's inner world connecting with their thoughts and feelings. While other media types rely primarily upon external cues to achieve this, the world of literature has the ability to take the receiver more directly into that person's world. Film and television, for example, provide glimpses of the inner world through facial gestures and expressiveness of speech, leaving the viewer in many instances to form their own interpretation of what a person's experience might be. Aspects such as frustration, rage or upset might be conveyed clearly enough although without all the intricacies and ambiguities of individual thoughts and feelings. The style of writing utilised (e.g. first or third person narrative) plays a significant role in the ways in which readers engage with the theme of mental illness and will be explored later in this chapter, paying particular attention to the type of relationship fostered, either of a connecting or distancing kind.

The themes of 'mental illness' or 'madness' have appeared within all the varied forms of writing (e.g. prose, poetry and drama) for thousands of years. The examples generally signify something of the varied societal attitudes relating to the historical era of their production. It is a popular choice of topic aided by the view that:

Portrayals of madness convey in symbolic form human beings'

preoccupation with their own mental functioning . . . in literature, as in daily life, madness is the perpetual amorphous threat within and the extreme of the unknown in fellow human beings.

(Feder 1980: 4)

The vast body of literature available to readers reflects the theme of mental illness from every conceivable angle ranging from negative, stigmatising types to positive, engaging ones. One appeal for writers concerning the inclusion of mental health content regards the enhanced degree of drama or spice that it lends to their narrative. It is something found in abundance within the horror and thriller genres, prolifically involving the full range of misleading and inaccurate stereotypes. Another attraction involving the more sensitive and informed writing concerns the author's desire to look specifically at the lived experience of mental health problems and to educate their readership accordingly.

Historical aspects

The medium of literature provides us with depictions of 'madness' that date back to the Ancient Roman and Greek writings of Homer and Virgil. The appeal of mental health content is reflected in Salkeld's statement that: 'Tales of madness are unsettling. They have a strange and enduring power to fascinate, amuse and appal beyond the limits of their own historical moment' (Salkeld 1993: 8). When reading texts from a different time, it is important to recognise something of the contextual views pertinent to the era of their publication. This means therefore utilising a 'historicist' approach as madness in ancient texts, for example, can only properly be understood by acknowledging ancient opinions about madness (Hershkowitz 1998).

Madness in Ancient Greek and Roman cultures was seen as the result of divine intervention or sickness (Padel 1995; Hershkowitz 1998). The Greek epics in particular portrayed the individual's struggle with various forms of trial while the tragedies dealt with passions and emotions of an *extreme kind*; fear, anger, hate, madness, jealousy and love in *extreme circumstances*; murder, suicide, incest, rape and mutilation (Barlow 1996). The belief that madness is caused and can only be cured by divine intervention continued to proliferate through the middle ages to the fourteenth and fifteenth centuries and included the views that madness resulted either in death and damnation or served as a test leading towards self-knowledge, confession and reform (Feder 1980). The combination of destructiveness and self-discovery-type messages are still evident within later centuries as illustrated within the dramatic work of Shakespeare. In *King Lear*, for example, the experience of madness provides the king with a new awareness of the suffering and injustice that can be found in society. Another common depiction within Shakespearian plays portrayed madness as a terrible and agonising experience of suffering.

The late eighteenth and nineteenth centuries included a number of extra-ordinarily popular stories about women who go mad when they lose their lovers. This represented a significant shift from the image of the madman in chains towards the woman whose insanity was regarded as an extension of her female condition (Small 1996). The depiction of 'mad woman' was also used in some instances to signify a destructive and malevolent background presence as illustrated with Mrs Danvers in Daphne de Maurier's *Rebecca* or Mrs Rochester in Charlotte Brontë's *Jane Eyre*.

The era of asylum care and incarceration provides some powerful examples such as *One Flew over the Cuckoo's Nest, Faces in the Water* and *The Bell Jar*. Interestingly, these accounts sit alongside the growing realisation that emerged in the late 1950s and early 1960s (Goffman 1961; Barton 1976; Scheff 1974) of the detrimental and depersonalising effects of institutional care. The trend of exploring expanded thought by authors such as Carlos Castaneda and Aldous Huxley helped to stimulate interest into the perceived world of altered cognition, although to a large extent this mirrored the trend for experimentation with drugs already being carried out by many in society. Lastly, the current era of community care and the greater visibility of mental health issues have contributed towards the steady increase in autobiographical first-person accounts concerning psychological distress that now feature regularly on best-selling lists.

Writer influences

The inclusion of mental health themes and content within written works is influenced significantly by the intention of the writer and may be the prime focus of the work or merely a part of the whole. The reasons why mental health content is addressed may be reflected in the type of narrative being written including:

- Autobiography (*what the act of writing gives to the author*)
  Deriving therapeutic value from the process of writing.
- Semi-autobiography (*what the experience of mental health problems gives to the art of writing*)
  Connectedness borne out of personal experience.
- Fiction (*what the inclusion of mental health material gives to the reader*)
  Lending dramatic impact to the narrative.

These three different types of writing offer a wide range of mental health perspectives. At one end of the spectrum we have the insightful, expressive and connected forms of writing that enable the reader to engage with those being depicted. At the other end we have the stereotypical and misleading portrayals where the driving factors of financial rewards and personal gain override other sensitivities.

Autobiography (therapeutic value)

To a certain degree autobiographical writing provides us with the most insightful and clear prose concerning issues of mental health. One might argue that it is the writing about 'mental illness' by those who best understand the material being handled. Although dating back over the centuries with examples such as George Trosse's *The Life of the Reverend Mr George Trosse* in 1693 and Bunyan's *Grace Abounding to the Chief of Sinners* in 1666, it is only over the past decade or so that there has been a significant increase in autobiographical writing centring upon personal distress and coping with traumatic experience. This type of writing has been notably gaining a greater acceptance in mainstream literature mirroring trends in society (e.g. the advent of community care) and its depiction within other media formats. It perhaps already has a proven track record in the popularity of many *coffee-table* magazines with their many varied stories of survival and coping with personal trauma. The need to understand, connect with or catch a glimpse of others' lives and problems, albeit a degree voyeuristically, appeals to a large number of the public. In contrast to the dramatic fictional portrayal, we have here the dramatic factual tale, in some cases every bit as suspenseful and compelling as their fictional counterparts. These publications include best-sellers and award winners such as David Solomon's (2002) *Noonday Demon: An Anatomy of Depression* (Mind book of the year 2002); Tim Lott's (1997) acclaimed *The Scent of Dried Roses* and the international best selling trilogy by Dave Pelzer (1995, 1997, 1999) of *A Child Called It, The Lost Boy* and *A Man Named Dave*.

Many of these accounts are both distressing as well as uplifting. In many cases they recount experiences of individuals who have endured a lifetime's suffering or, because of certain life events, have hit rock bottom, survived and dragged themselves back up. A notable example is the book *Addicted* by the footballer Tony Adams (1998) which recounts his recovery from alcoholism. Within the plethora of footballer autobiographies this one carries comments such as: 'So good, so scorchingly honest and revealing . . .'; and 'An impressive and candid memoir . . . it's hard to recall another book in which the author has spoken with such self-lacerating honesty.' It is a painfully honest account of his personal fragmentation although provides a very strong sense of connecting with a real person. A less honest narrative, for example a more typically macho account, would lose much of this book's very real appeal.

A major influencing factor concerning this type of writing concerns the therapeutic value afforded both the author from the process of writing and the reader from the sharing of their experience. A significant part of the process for the author is in the working through and making sense of traumatic experience. This is clearly illustrated by Anne Deveson in her account *Tell Me I'm Here*, relating to her search for a cure and understanding for her schizophrenic son through his illness and ultimately his suicide:

I needed to write this book: to lay before myself the richness of the experience and the bleakness. I needed not to deny the bad aspects because these were a part of the whole and, for me, serenity rests in the whole. I still feel distress when I think of the terrors that Jonathan endured. I miss him. But I no longer feel despair.

(Deveson 1992: 259)

A sense of resolution and acceptance is also illustrated by Tim Lott in *A Scent of Dried Roses*. This book attempts to make sense of and understand both his mother's suicide and his own feelings of depression. He concludes that he subsequently feels detached from suffocating feelings of guilt and:

I cannot ever know if I am guilty, but if I am, I no longer have difficulty forgiving myself, I have decided that I would rather not be such a supernaturally good person – as my mother fantasised herself, finally to be, that it involves me killing myself, or living a life of despair, in order to prove it.

(Lott 1997: 263)

Similarly, David Pelzer's trilogy beginning with the book *A Child Called It* can be seen as a search for understanding and reconciling his own experience of being abused and neglected as a child. He writes about horrific cruelty from the perspective of a survivor although with a healthy and positive outlook for the future.

The steady increase in autobiographical work concerning mental health issues is complemented by publishers such as Chipmunkapublishing, whose core purpose is to publish work by individuals who have experienced or been touched by mental distress. Two of their publications in particular continue the writing as therapy theme. Jason Pegler, commenting upon writing about his experience of manic depression (*A Can of Madness*), said: 'Writing saved my life. It was the only way that I could rationally come to terms with the humiliation that I felt from being labelled with a mental illness' (Pegler 2003: 31).

Likewise, another author, Dolly Sen, stated about the writing of *The World is Full of Laughter*, a book about her experience of depression: 'I say of my book that it started out as a suicide note and ended as a celebration of life . . . for me creativity gave me control in a world where because of a diagnosis, I had no control' (Sen 2003: 31).

The *writing as therapy* theme is certainly one that needs encouragement and avenues for further development. Indeed, many mental health promotional initiatives such as that run by Leeds Mind (*Including Us*) encourage writing as a means of expression and sharing. The main strength of this process is the opportunity for making sense of personal experience and gaining a degree of resolution and control over one's life. It aids the process of survival and the act of writing itself allows the author to ventilate and share their thoughts and feelings initially in a way that feels safe. What perhaps is unclear is the degree of guidance or pressure that those writing such accounts might feel under, particularly with the commercial value of highly traumatic and distressing revelations proving so attractive to publishers and readers alike.

Autobiographical accounts by celebrities proliferate and fill the best-seller shelves of bookshops. They are written with wide-ranging degrees of skill and ability, some apparently very hurriedly to meet public demand. Some of these include accounts of dealing with mental health issues, for example Geri Halliwell's (2003) *Just for the Record*, Robbie Williams' (2002) *Somebody Someday* and Paul Gascoigne's (2005) *Gazza: My Story*. An interesting account is provided by the accomplished New Zealand writer Janet Frame with her book *An Angel at My Table*. This publication details her treatment and hospitalisation for mental health problems including her fortunate reprieve from psychosurgery. It is notable that critical receipt of this work centred upon the 'autobiographical' label as reducing the impact of the book's intellectual content as it emphasised her experience more than her ideas (Unsworth 1995). This is an extremely restrictive viewpoint that diminishes the powerful and connecting nature of this expressive and highly insightful narrative.

What is interesting today is the widening appeal and accessibility of autobiographical writing, a form of expression that was previously conceived as the lifetime reflections of highly prominent individuals (Chamberlain and Thompson 1998). This genre has now widened to encompass previously unknown authors who have 'a story to tell'. Celebrity writers are more commonly found within mainstream publishing and are helping to lead the way in making this form of narrative more acceptable and accessible. It even includes collaborative works that marry the credibility and authority of mental health professionals with the popular appeal of noted celebrities such as *Depression and How to Survive It* (Spike Milligan/Anthony Clare 1994) and *Families and How to Survive Them* (Robin Skynner/John Cleese 1993). The professional voice adds a further dimension here and Professor Kay Jamison's (1997) excellent autobiographical account (*An Unquiet Mind*) of her own battles with manic-depression presents an insightfully written account supported by clear scientific evidence.

For the reader, the attraction of this type of work may be generated either by curiosity or a desire to achieve a sense of connectedness and identification with the mental health experience. As Miller (2002) illustrates, the proximity of shared experience might apply where an individual reads a text and feels that it has been written especially for them. This highlights a self-help feature of many of these accounts whereby readers gain a sense of shared experience as well as a degree of hope and optimism through another's narrative. The point at which they are written is important as they generally reflect a picture of survival and resolution, not one of hopelessness and unresolved conflict. Nonetheless they are not necessarily easy to read and the awfulness and distress of what is being narrated can be unbearable at times; for example, the tormenting cruelty suffered by David Pelzer as a child at the hands of his abusive, alcoholic mother and his neglecting, ignorant father.

The rather astonishing popularity of this genre of writing is illustrated by their regularly featuring within top-selling book lists. A recent glance at the *Sunday Times* (13 February 2005) best-selling non-fiction book list illustrates this point with the top two selling hardback books *A Brother's Journey* by Richard Pelzer and *The Little Prisoner* by Jane Elliott, both being about childhood abuse. Similarly, the 'top ten' paperback list contained five such entries that included:

- *Sickened* / Julie Gregory (Munchausen's by proxy)
- *One Child* / Torey Hayden (childhood abuse – a biographical account written by a therapist)
- *The Privilege of Youth* / Dave Pelzer (childhood abuse)
- *To Die For* / Carol Lee (anorexia)
- *My Story* / Dave Pelzer (childhood abuse)

These types of narrative are obviously extremely popular and it is unclear as to the types of pressure or coercion that might be exerted upon authors to include material they feel uneasy or uncertain about revealing. Also uncertain is the extent to which the commercial value of these products plays a part in their writing. Richard Pelzer's *A Brother's Journey*, for example, was written following his brother David's astonishing success with his series of auto-biographical works detailing childhood abuse. While in all probability having his own reasons for writing this book there is perhaps the danger of commercial considerations overtaking those of therapeutic ones. Nevertheless, the valuable sense of exposure cannot be overestimated especially where taboo topics such as child abuse are brought out of the shadows and into the public arena thereby enabling others so affected to feel encouraged about expressing and sharing their own experiences.

Semi-autobiography (connectedness)

> When a writer draws on his own experience of insanity as the subject or emotional source of his work, what is of most interest is his adaptation of delusion, dissociation, or other aberrations to the creation of a unique view of his society, his art and his own mind.
>
> (Feder 1980: 9)

Clearly, experience of mental distress provides authors with a degree of expression both useful in writing directly about that experience or using it as a base from which to draw upon. Themes of personal trauma, distress or difficulty are written about with greater insight and are more elaborately and expressively laid down in the main text. In a sense, one's own personal experience breathes life into the body of writing. This approach to writing is regarded as semi-autobiographical and has many examples within classical and contemporary literature. Perhaps the earliest clear example is Goethe's *The Sorrows of Young Werther* (*Die Leiden des Jungen Werthers*) which was originally published in 1774. This piece of writing is modelled upon Goethe's own personal experience of frustrated love as well as the suicide of his close friend Karl Wilhelm Jerusalem. It is very vivid and expressive prose describing how Werther is progressively driven to more fevered and tortured thoughts of despair because of an unattainable love, longing for suicide as his only release. The power of this piece of work and the degree to which readers identified with Goethe's Werther is illustrated in the outcry which followed its publication with assertions that it led a number of people to take their own lives. The increased rate in suicide across Europe following its publication saw the book banned in a number of countries (Pirkis and Blood 2001).

There may be a contrast between semi-autobiographical writing and autobiographical in terms of the author's intention and the resultant impact their work has upon them. In some cases it seems the art of writing is an all-consuming process that has a destructive effect upon the author. Consigning one's emotions into written words can, as has been addressed above, leave some with a feeling of resolution and clarity although at the same time can leave others drained and spent, having given all for their art. Two prominent names in the world of literature who are recognised as 'suffering through their art' are Sylvia Plath and Malcolm Lowry. Sylvia Plath committed suicide a few months after the publication of *The Bell Jar*, a piece of work directly related to her own illness and experience of mental health treatment. It is a piece of writing rich in prose, symbolism and imagery, all of which can be traced directly back to Plath's own mental anguish. The sense of creative expression being borne out of inner torment is related by her former husband, the poet Ted Hughes who states: 'The root system of her talent was a deep and inclusive inner crisis . . . She used details from [her outer upheavals and her preoccupation] as a matter of course for images to develop her X-Rays' (Hughes 1985). The essence here is the direct channel provided between the author's own felt experience of distress and the words which are subsequently placed down on paper.

Another author who is regarded as writing from personal experience is the writer Malcolm Lowry. *Under the Volcano* (1947), widely regarded as his best work, is a semi-autobiographical novel with the main character Geoffrey Firmin's destructive alcoholism mirroring Lowry's own. The many links with Lowry's own life include alcoholism, depression, murderous attacks on his wife and a number of suicide attempts before his eventual death after a drinking bout (Bradbrook 1974). Lowry's own experience no doubt provided a rich depth of understanding that is reflected within the narrative itself. There is a hallucinatory quality to the writing borne out in a narrative style that is full of symbolism and metaphor. Grace (1982) regards the writing of this book, which took ten years to complete, as having a detrimental impact upon its author, exhausting his genius in the creation of a single masterpiece, his other fiction being neglected and relatively unknown.

> Indeed the words of Lowry himself in the short poem '*After publication of Under the Volcano*' supports this. Commencing with the line: 'success is like some horrible disaster,' he continues to elaborate upon the damaging toll exacted upon himself through stark terms such as ruination and damnation. He finishes the poem by rueing the sense of acclaim afforded this publication and wishing that he had been '. . . left in darkness forever to founder and fail'.
>
> (Birney 1962).

Another writer worthy of a mention here includes the New Zealand writer Janet Frame whose experience is very different from that of Lowry and Plath as she regarded writing as a way to survive (Hannah 1978). She has written a number of books which are clearly in part informed through her own experiences of mental health problems such as *Faces in the Water, Scented Gardens for the Blind* and *Owls do Cry*. In particular, many parallels have been drawn between her own experience within psychiatric hospitals and those of Istina Mavet, the principal character in her novel *Faces in the Water* (Ferrier 1995), although Janet Frame herself refutes suggestions that it is directly about her but under a different name (Penny 1992). Where writing has a strong foundation within direct experience the distinction between fiction and reality is not always easy to define as some of the imagery and messages being presented can be extremely persuasive. For example, a degree of alarm was caused by the widespread belief that Frame's *Owls do Cry* was an autobiographical account, in response to which she managed to convince a doctor, who had read the book, that this was not so by demonstrating the absence of leucotomy scars. As she aptly summed up: 'Not every aspiring writer has such a terrifying but convincing method of displaying to others "proof" that she has been writing fiction' (Bruce 1975: 148).

A core component therefore of the semi-autobiographical category relates to the fact that despite the strength and expressiveness of this form of writing, there can be very different consequences for the writer, with some finding it a painful and consuming process whereas others feel liberated and supported by it.

Fiction (dramatic impact)

There is little doubt that mental health issues have a curiosity appeal and can be compelling for the reader of literature. They add a degree of attractiveness that may be intentionally or unintentionally manipulated in order to engage the reader. This voyeuristic quality is not too dissimilar to the historical pastime of visiting psychiatric institutions where madness was presented as the prime exhibit. It is, as Ingram (1991) asserts, the dramatic equivalent of the literary or actual sightseeing tour of lunacy. Adding mental health themes to a narrative may be seen as a purposeful attempt at manipulating the reader's engagement with the material accessed. It may be the subject which sells the book or which helps to maintain focus where interest may be flagging. From an attentional perspective, influential factors include stimuli that are novel, engage curiosity and stand out by virtue of their intensity (Child 2004), all of which are stimulated by the inclusion of mental health content. These lend products a touch of drama and impact, serving to draw the reader in and to keep them engaged. Wally Lamb's book *I Know This Much is True* (2000), for example, commences with Dominick Birdsey's schizophrenic twin brother cutting off his hand in a public library as a result of delusional thought processes. This occurs right at the beginning of a fairly long publication (912 pages) and serves to instantly engage the reader and hook them into the narrative. What follows, though, is a degree of more sensitive writing detailing the impact that mental illness has upon a family.

A consequence of the significant impact created by mental health content is the potential for wide-ranging exposure and enhancing the popularity of books that perhaps would not otherwise gain as wide a circulation. Selling books and reaching a wide audience is good when the messages being transmitted are positive and sensitive. The problem lies, however, in the wealth of popular literature that sensationalises mental health issues and which is often misleading and inaccurate. In order to look at the fictional representation it is perhaps a useful exercise to compare the handling of particular themes within different literary genres. For the purposes of this comparison, the topic of child abuse will be looked at as portrayed by Virginia Andrews' (1979) fictional novel *Flowers in the Attic* and David Pelzer's (1995) autobiographical narrative *A Child Called It*. Although based upon a similar theme, the way in which this extremely delicate topic has been handled and the overall message being transmitted is vastly different. Pelzer's account is much more sensitively handled and portrays an overall message of survival and hope, whereas *Flowers in the Attic* seems more interested in dramatically engaging its readers with its bleak message of destruction. Unlike *A Child Called It*, the fictional narrative is written from a position of bitterness and a desire for revenge. It is unforgiving in tone:

> I find every word I put down, I put down with tears, with bitter blood, with sour gall, well mixed and blended with shame and guilt ... The tempest of rage that once stormed within me has simmered down so I can write I hope with truth and with less hatred and prejudice.
>
> (Andrews 1979: 7)

The message throughout the book is one of destructiveness and pain, the surviving characters leaving the house of their confinement battered and seeking revenge. In contrast to this, Pelzer's autobiographical account is optimistic and hopeful despite the appalling nature of some of the experiences being related and at the end of the book he writes: 'I believe it is important for people to know that no matter what lies in their past, they can overcome the dark side and press on to a brighter world' (Pelzer 1995: 145). He also goes on to describe the supportive and healthy relationship he has with his son and his hope for the future. It is a book that has been written with forgiveness and understanding and with a clear indication that the cycle of child abuse can be broken, unlike that of the tale being told by *Flowers in the Attic* and its sequels where the cycle of abuse is perpetuated. Although the packaging of these books obviously changes with subsequent reprints, they are still significantly different in overall appearance. With regard to the editions accessed, *A Child Called It* is very simply presented with a bright, white cover featuring a black and white photo of an innocent-looking young child. It is appealing in a way that is starkly different from that of *Flowers in the Attic* which is synonymous with many horror books with its dark, Gothic style cover displaying a pair of haunted-looking eyes gazing out over the top of a shadowy silhouetted mansion. What is evident from both of these publication types is that the fictional version appears primarily concerned with a dramatic engagement of readers and a selling of books rather than in showing any real sensitivity towards the topic concerned. The autobiographical account, on the other hand, demonstrates a greater concern about the overall message and the support and help that can be gained by others reading it.

Perhaps the most negative and careless mental health references are made within the genre of horror or thriller writing. While a good deal of these seem to pay little obvious attention to actual facts, others achieve a blend of drama and impact along with a more thoughtful exploration of themes, for example *The Wasp Factory* or *American Psycho*. A common representation within the fictional domain is the mentally ill killer whose portrayal, as illustrated by Thomas Harris's Hannibal Lecter character, seems rarely true to life. This characterisation, according to Ressler and Schachtman (1992), combines attributes of several different sorts of killers, with a range of personality dynamics that would be highly unlikely to coexist in any one person in the real world. It is borne out by Wahl's (1995) assertion that, despite their apparent popularity, the psychotic psychopath is a very unrealistic and misleading characterisation. It is a compelling one, though, and one that proliferates in numerous accounts by popular writers within this genre (e.g. Patricia Cornwell) wherein accuracy is displaced by the need for exciting and dramatic prose. An interesting example, however, is demonstrated by Jeffery Deaver's *Praying for Sleep*, a thriller about a schizophrenic man who has escaped from a hospital for the criminally insane and is apparently pursuing the woman who testified against him. This novel cleverly uses the public's inaccurate understanding and preconditioned feelings about the mentally ill to deliver its biggest surprise at the end of this work when it is revealed that he is actually completely innocent of all the violent crimes attributed to him. These revelations cause the character to undergo a complete transformation in the eyes of the reader from a dangerous and clever manipulator to a vulnerable and caring person.

Regulation and censorship

Literature unlike other media sources such as the press or television has far fewer restrictions or regulations governing what is presented. There is a fair deal of freedom presented to authors in what can be written although some degree of restriction or censorship is imposed by the publishers or external organisations. It is normally left to individual publishers to review work prior to its publication and place restrictions where it is deemed necessary in order to comply with governmental legislation and specific acts concerned with copyright, defamation, racism and sexism, disability, human rights and obscene publications.

Some notable publications have met with fierce condemnation from various groups and have had various sanctions placed upon them. In September 2002, the publisher Gallimard bowed to legal threats and decided not to resupply bookshops with *Rose Bonbon* by Nicolas Jones-Gorlin, the story of a murderous paedophile. Another novel, *Satanic Verses*, earned its author Salman Rushdie a *fatwa* (death sentence) from the Ayatollah Khomeini in Iran. While censorship is geared towards restricting publication there are notable examples where the opposite has happened, such as in the case of D.H. Lawrence's *Lady Chatterley's Lover*, which sold 200,000 copies in a day following Penguin's triumph following its acquittal from prosecution under the Obscene Publications Act. An important aspect regarding censorship relates to the organisation or group imposing sanctions and it is normally the view of a group that holds overall power and influence which determines what is deemed acceptable or not. In some cases this is deemed a protective measure, generally agreed upon and supported by the majority of people. Alternatively, it might be viewed as a means of stifling individual expression, something that is enforced through extreme measures. There are many historical examples of this with authors forced to write in exile, their writing deemed unacceptable in their own country, for example the Russian authors Solzhenitsyn (*Gulag Archipelago*) and Boris Pasternak (*Doctor Zhivago*).

The censorship argument with books generally relates to what is deemed unacceptable by certain groups or societies. Clearly this may differ from one individual or culture to another and what tends to matter is how powerful the dissenting voice is. Traditionally, the mentally ill have been poorly represented and have been given little *voice* with which to make their displeasure known. Currently, a number of mental health service-user groups are taking a much more active stance with media providers in terms of collaboration, campaigning and offering feedback. The difficulty with the medium of literature is the huge wealth of existing literature of a stigmatising kind already in circulation, including well-established or critically well-received texts as well as books that have enjoyed a huge commercial appeal. In order for censorship to be applied properly to the stigmatisation of mental illness, there needs to be a consensus from a powerful enough collective voice that such stigmatisation is deemed unacceptable. Although the newsprint and broadcast media have come under significant scrutiny from mental health advocates it seems that in the world of literature, with a few minor exceptions, little has been done.

Riddell (2002) argues that while there is a place for regulation in the arts, censorship does not take account of readers' ability to detach themselves from what they are reading, and the fact that they are not all impressionable people easily swayed by what they encounter. It may be true to a point that reading about violence or self-destructiveness does not necessarily influence one's own personal behaviour. The continued reinforcement of stereotypical mental health content, however, has an insidious effect upon the public who may have limited access to more productive and accurate material. Because of the difficulties in restricting the negative portrayals of mental health themes it seems that the best counter is provided through education. This in particular helps individuals to understand what they are reading and to discriminate better between positive and negative messages located within a narrative. It is greatly helped by autobiographical work and initiatives that promote and celebrate positive mental health writing such as the Mind book awards that identify some of the best texts covering mental health themes with previous winners including David Solomon's (2002) factual/ autobiographical text on depression (*The Noonday Demon*) and Bernlef's (1988) first-person narrative detailing the experience of a man with dementia (*Out of Mind*).

The 'inner world' (*inside looking out*)

One of the most powerful aspects of literature is its ability to travel with significant depth into the 'inner world' of characters and directly connect with another's thoughts and feelings, seeing the world from their perspective. It is a process of identification where we might develop a sense of connectedness with others and for a while suspend our own lives and travel with them along the particular journey they are taking. The main style of writing providing this type of direct contact is the use of first-person narrative. It can help by taking the reader directly into the fragmented and confused thought processes experienced within a number of acute mental health states and thereby prove an enlightening and educating experience, helping to develop one's sensitivity towards those experiencing mental health problems. It can also, though, be an immensely discomforting and scary process as felt, for example, when the experience of a person's ordered world becomes more chaotic and fragmented. An example of this can be seen in Hannah Green's *I Never Promised You a Rose Garden*:

> She saw the doctor's mouth moving, and imagined that it was spewing

questions and accusations. She began to fall, going with Anterrabae through his fire-fragmented darkness into Yr. This time the fall was far. There was utter darkness for a long time and then a greyness, seen only in bands across the eye. The place was familiar; it was the pit. In this place gods and Collect moaned and shouted, but even they were unintelligible. Human sounds came, too, but they came without meaning. The world intruded, but it was a shattered world and unrecognisable.

(Green 1964: 34)

Reading through this passage and others in the book we are given a very strong sense of Deborah's feelings of disassociation, anxiety and powerlessness. This perspective (*inside looking out*) is uniquely different from the external one which might describe a person's odd behaviour without the reader gaining any sense or understanding as to what is going on within.

Connecting with an individual's felt experience can be related to the psychotherapeutic term empathy, which is regarded as the ability to sense another person's world as if it were one's own (Rogers 1951; Cassedy and Cutliffe 1998). From a therapeutic perspective, a potential problem within this process involves the therapist having too great an emotional reaction and subsequently moving away psychologically from their client (Gladstein 1983). If this is true then of the trained therapist, it is highly likely that the reader will also experience significant problems in connecting with distressing and uncomfortable emotions. An important issue here relates to the fact that readers will differ in their ability or even their desire to get closer to certain characters encountered within literature. This is perhaps true with Doris Lessing's *Briefing for a Descent into Hell* where the text itself is extremely difficult to stay with. The book's narrative focuses primarily upon the fragmented and confused thoughts of Charles Watkins and is written in a largely unstructured and rambling prose, occasionally 'surfacing' to catch fragments of dialogue before again returning to his delusional world. As the story progresses, the narrative becomes more ordered and less chaotic. Sentences become generally shorter than those that at times last for a number of pages and the content becomes more tuned into the prime character's surroundings, noticing more of the world outside of his internal one. It is a strongly and creatively written piece of work that depicts very vividly the feelings of disconnectedness and confused thought processes operating within certain psychotic states. The form of expression conveyed here is reflected in other examples that also use what could be described as the language of madness. Publications such as these lend a degree of credibility to the expression by those deemed to be mentally ill and include some notable examples including Jonathan Swift's (1704) *Tale of a Tub*, a narrative that gradually reveals the fact that the narrator was once an inmate of Bedlam (Hawes 1996), and *Lucida Intervalla*, James Carkesse's 1679 text that is perhaps the first collection of verse published in England by an inmate of an asylum. Accounts such as these have helped to develop a new climate of expressive communication and, as Maclennan (1992) highlights, allow the experience of madness to become available in literature for the production and expression of subjective meaning.

The disturbing nature of remaining within the direct world of madness is perhaps aptly illustrated by the novel *American Psycho* which provides the reader with an insightful yet unsettling connection with the thoughts of a psychopathic killer. Patrick Bateman's sense of emptiness and cold detachment is aptly illustrated by the first-person narrative used and the reader is maintained throughout the book at a disturbingly close proximity to the inner world of this killer as he emotionlessly dispatches victim after victim. His only real sense of insight is acknowledged towards the end of the book, as shown in the following passage:

> There is no real me, only an entity, something illusory, and though I can hide my cold gaze and you can shake my hand and feel flesh gripping yours and maybe you can even sense our lifestyles are comparable : I am simply not there . . . my conscience, my pity, my hopes disappeared a long time ago if they ever did exist . . . my pain is constant and sharp and I do not hope for a better world for anyone. In fact I want my pain to be inflicted on others. I want no one to escape.
>
> (Easton-Ellis 1991: 377)

This book provides an unsettling experience for the reader and it is at times extremely difficult to stay with, perhaps more so because we are led towards an unfamiliar vantage point. Our perspective within horror or thriller books is normally somewhere close to the thoughts and feelings of the person being pursued. This text connects us with the inner world of the predator allowing the reader to see not only the horror of his actions but also the horror of his thoughts. The way in which these types of work are handled and the opportunity to educate the public as to the 'greater picture' is important because of the tendency to stereotype and apply isolated examples to the entire collective known as 'the mentally ill'.

First- versus third-person narrative

Genette (1980) identifies two main types of writing: external focalisation, where the recounting is carried out by an observer focusing on a character, and internal focalisation where a narrative is told through the consciousness of a character. These narrative styles (in essence third and first person) lead the reader into very different relationships with the characters being portrayed and strongly influence the sense of identification and connectedness they have with them. This is outlined by Lothe (2000) who indicates that within first-person narratives the reader is active within the plot as opposed to third-person writing of being located outside or above it. An example of the significance of this can be illustrated by the following two extracts taken from Mary Shelley's (1818) *Frankenstein* and J.K. Rowling's (2000) *Harry Potter and the Goblet of Fire*.

- Internal focalisation – *Frankenstein*:

They are kind – they are the most excellent creatures in the world; but unfortunately they are prejudiced against me. I have good dispositions; my life has been hitherto harmless and in some degree beneficial; but a fatal prejudice clouds their eyes, and where they ought to see a feeling and kind friend they behold a detestable monster.

The old man [replied] . . . 'I am blind but cannot judge of your countenance, but there is something in your words which persuades me you are sincere.'

. . . At that instant the cottage door was opened, and Felix, Safie and Agatha entered. Who can describe their horror and consternation on beholding me? Agatha fainted, and Safie unable to attend to her friend, rushed out the cottage. Felix darted forward and with supernatural force tore me from his father, to whose knees I could have torn him limb from limb, as the lion rends the antelope. But my heart sunk within me as with bitter sickness, and I refrained . . .

. . . Cursed, cursed creator! Why did I live? Why I that instant, did I not extinguish the spark of existence which you had so wantonly bestowed? I know not: despair had not yet taken possession of me; my feelings were those of rage and revenge. I could with pleasure have destroyed the cottage and its inhabitants, and have glutted myself with their shrieks and misery.

(Shelley 1818)

- External focalisation – *Harry Potter and the Goblet of Fire* (2000), 'The madness of Mr Crouch':

Next moment a man had staggered out from behind a tall oak. For a moment, Harry didn't recognise him . . . then he realised it was Mr Crouch. He looked as though he had been travelling for days. The knees of his robes were ripped and bloody; his face scratched; he was unshaven and grey with exhaustion. His neat hair and moustache were both in need of a wash and a trim. His strange appearance, however, was nothing to the way he was behaving. Muttering and gesticulating, Mr Crouch appeared to be talking to someone that he alone could see. He reminded Harry vividly of an old tramp he had seen once when out shopping with the Dursleys. That man, too, had been conversing wildly with thin air . . . 'I've done . . . stupid . . . thing . . .' Mr Crouch breathed. He looked utterly mad. His eyes were rolling and bulging, and a trickle of spittle was sliding down his chin.

(Rowling 2000)

The first extract from Mary Shelley's classic text depicts the creature's sense of longing for companionship. It is essentially the tale of a child who wants to be loved but instead receives rejection and abuse, subsequently becoming rejecting and abusive towards others. The impact upon the reader can be seen as being in stark contrast to the following extract that presents a very different message with phrases such as: 'He [Mr Crouch] looked utterly mad'. Mr Crouch no doubt presents his observers with a similarly foreboding appearance to that of the creature as seen by Felix, Safie and Agatha. We are not given the benefit here of accessing Mr Crouch's thoughts and perhaps experiencing some of his fear and confusion. Instead, he is presented as an image of unpredictability and somebody from whom we might seek to distance ourselves. This latter extract portrays the stereotypical view of madness being a visible entity, borne out by Mr Crouch's responding to voices, facial grimaces and his overall state of dishevelment. A core difference therefore between these examples is the vantage point from which each person is viewed. With Mr Crouch, we are located on the *outside looking in*, registering from the same perspective as Harry Potter, his wild behaviour and unkempt appearance. With the first extract, however, we are on the *inside looking out*, gaining a sense of connection with the creature's inner world and as a consequence responding in a different way to the cottage's inhabitants who see a monster instead of a being in need of loving care. As with Jastrow's duck/rabbit image (see Figure 4.1), our understanding of what we are exposed to can change dramatically if looked at from an alternative perspective. The important point perhaps concerns the degree to which readers are actually alerted to the presence of an alternative viewpoint. From a mental health perspective the significance is in recognising the person who exists within a condition or diagnosis, and reflecting the person-centred approach as advocated strongly through the humanist school (Rogers 1961; Maslow 1971). Essentially, the more that individuals are able to connect with and understand another's felt experience regarding mental health issues, the more they will be able to challenge and question common stereotypes, starting to see the person in a new and more productive light.

Survival versus destruction

The portrayal of mental health content in literature covers a wide spectrum that can be seen as lying on a continuum somewhere between the polarised positions of *survival* and *destruction*. The *survival* category demonstrates an ability to cope with mental health problems and offers hope whereas the *destruction* one portrays various conditions as all-consuming and destructive for self or others.

Survival

This category focuses upon mental illness as a survivable condition and features strongly throughout autobiographical accounts as well as within a range of fictional narratives. The main message being conveyed here regards individuals developing ways of coping with various mental health conditions, aided in part by support from others and particular treatments offered. The primary messages are those of re-emergence from one's struggles with mental health difficulties as well as learning to live with and accept them. These accounts are to a large degree inspirational and heartening, providing the reader with a sense of hope and optimism relating to specific psychological difficulties. This message is strongly demonstrated in Janet Fitch's (1999) *White Oleander*, a book that relates the tale of a young girl, Astrid, and her search for meaning in her life following a series of rejections and abuse as well as her mother's imprisonment. It conveys very powerfully her ability to overcome extreme physical and emotional trauma through her incredibly strong will to survive. Another novel, *I Know This Much Is True* (Lamb 2000), shifts the attention onto family members and reflects upon how they learn to cope with their own feelings of helplessness and suffocating feelings of guilt. It is a sensitively written narrative that strongly conveys the impact that mental illness has upon the whole family as well as the support mechanisms used by them to cope.

Examples of individuals re-emerging from a distorted state can be found as far back as the Ancient Greek times as illustrated in the tale of Heracles' awakening following his murderous rage:

> Ah, I am still breathing and I see all I should see, the sky, the earth and the sun's shafts. I was swamped somehow by a terrible confusion of mind and my breath comes hot and unsteady from my lungs, not calm at all. But look, why am I anchored like a ship with ropes around my powerful chest and arms? Why am I sitting against the broken stone pillar with corpses all around me? . . . Is there some friend of mine anywhere who could cure my ignorance?
>
> (Simon 1978: 99)

This example depicts the picture of Heracles' distorted cognitive state being transient in nature showing him becoming lucid and aware of his surroundings even though he is in this instance greeted with the appalling consequences of his actions. While a renewed sense of clarity is met here with despair, many other accounts portray a different picture, that of awakening to the joys of life as shown in Tim Lott's autobiographical novel *The Scent of Dried Roses*:

> I begin to take them [anti-depressant medication] every day. I have absolutely no faith that they will work. . . . Since the tablets supposedly take

> three weeks to work, that day I estimate will be 28 December 1987 . . .
> [On] 28 December I awake, unusually first thing in the morning. I am
> alone. I have an odd perception. There is a pigeon cooing on the balcony
> outside my bedroom window. It is pleasant and soothing. I haven't
> noticed birdsong for a long time . . . I feel strange in that I feel normal,
> average . . . As if by magic, all my thoughts about sin and redemption,
> God and the devil, have disappeared. It occurs to me that the desire to
> kill myself is utterly ridiculous. Why would I want to kill myself? I know,
> quite clearly and calmly now, like a camera suddenly finding focus, that I
> really have been ill, and equally that I have begun to recover.
>
> (Lott 1997: 245)

The message of re-emergence is similarly covered in other narratives such
as Sylvia Nasar's (1998) biographical account (*A Beautiful Mind*) of the
gifted mathematician John Nash and his survival from a debilitating set of
experiences with schizophrenia. Nash's recovery is topped off in the fairy-tale
style of triumph over adversity through being awarded the Nobel Prize for his
seminal work with game theory.

The concept of survival is heavily featured within the autobiographical
novel with numerous examples now available involving those that centre upon
an individual's personal experience or others that feature a shared collective
trauma. The collective accounts are written by individuals about experiences
that are shared such as social deprivation, poverty or political oppression. A
number of examples can be illustrated here including the book *Angela's
Ashes* which portrays Frank McCourt's astonishing ability to emerge from
what reads as an appalling catalogue of tragedy and hardship (McCourt
1996). Another account, Alexander Solzhenitsyn's (1963) *One Day in the Life
of Ivan Denisovich*, conveys a message familiar to a number of people struggling with conditions such as alcoholism or depression; that of coping 'one
day at a time'. This narrative centres upon life in a Siberian labour camp and
the way in which the central character and others discover various means to
survive within the stark and punishing hardships they have to endure. Perhaps a more astonishing account is written by Tadeusz Borowski (1959), an
Auschwitz survivor whose book *This Way for the Gas, Ladies and Gentleman*
demonstrates the will to survive (mainly through numbness and detachment)
found among those who had to endure the unendurable. This does not mean
to say that they are able to actually overcome such trauma, a point aptly
illustrated by the author's suicide in 1951. Lastly, there are a number of
excellent accounts detailing the experience of living through Chairman
Mao's cultural revolution in China including Jung Chan's *Wild Swans* and
Hong Ying's *Daughter of the River*. These books aptly sum up the restrictive-
ness, fear and privations that formed part of daily life, although also illustrate
the determination and strength found by many to overcome these and survive.

The steady increase in written accounts reflecting the survivable side of
mental health difficulties or psychological trauma is both positive and

encouraging. The popularity of these types of account is perhaps reflected in the *human interest* theme (Cortazzi 1993), although we can also consider the dramatic nature of the tale being recounted. It seems as if the greatest impact is created where a person's suffering seems unimaginable yet a will to survive still exists. The appeal that these types of narrative have for publishers and readers alike does present a problem in that what might be regarded as more 'ordinary' accounts of mental illness are consequently not as sought after. What is needed perhaps are avenues for airing experiences of coping with mental health problems that do not need to involve the worst forms of trauma or distress and are also representative of large numbers of people who are not at present being covered.

Destructiveness

The theme of destructiveness with regard to mental illness can be looked at from a number of perspectives involving negative consequences for the persons concerned or for those around them. The 'violence to others' view is perhaps the more popular and one that unsettles the reader especially when linked to accounts that portray victims as innocent and unsuspecting. It is the random and unpredictable nature of many of the portrayed attacks and the victim's complete innocence and vulnerability that make these more frightening to readers, raising the idea that the sporadic violence of madmen can reach anyone, even people like them (Wahl 1995). The degree of drama and suspense related here make mental illness as a theme a very appealing and attractive choice for writers. Indeed, books about psychopathic killers such as Thomas Harris' series of books about Hannibal Lecter, Bret Easton-Ellis' *American Psycho* and Iain Banks' *The Wasp Factory* have all proven extraordinarily popular

The *destructiveness to self* theme is aptly conveyed either directly as a consequence of a person's mental health difficulties or as a process visited on them by others. The former demonstrates the negative and all-consuming nature of a person's condition which they are unable to cope with or overcome. One example of this is provided by Malcolm Lowry's (1947) *Under the Volcano* which deals with the subject of alcoholism and the principal character Geoffrey Firmin's progressive absorption within a world of despair, resignation and isolation. Despite the available care and support of his wife Yvonne and friend Hugh, he is unable to help himself or take heart from their optimism and concern, instead feeling contemptible and unworthy. The narrative follows his progressive downward spiral through his steady absorption with alcohol, alienation from those who care for him, defilement with a prostitute and eventual death.

The sense of destruction, as briefly alluded to above, is something that can be visited upon an individual by other people. This is portrayed within a number of texts as a consequence of the controlling and abusive regime of care encountered. Perhaps the most well-known account of this is Ken

Kesey's *One Flew over the Cuckoo's Nest* that viewed the needs and interests of the institution coming firmly before those of the patients, and where non-compliance was treated brutally and harshly. The overriding sense of power-lessness and impotence experienced by those who are mentally ill is also illustrated in other accounts such as Janet Frame's *Faces in the Water* show-ing patients waiting meekly and passively for treatments such as ECT. This process is taken a stage further in Marge Piercy's *Woman on the Edge of Time* with an illustration of the terrifying concept of social control:

> 'That's Alice Blue Bottom,' Sybil hissed. 'Look what they've done to her!'
> 'What is it? Did she have an accident ?' ... 'It looks like they busted her head. Maybe she tried to get away.'
> ... Skip shook his head 'They did a kind of operation. They stuck needles in her brain.'
> ... Connie called out 'Is it true you got needles stuck in your ... head?'
> 'No lie electrodes they call them'
> '... Alice, if they're electrodes where are the wires?' Sybil asked cautiously.
> 'You old fashion. No wires. They use a little radio, and they stick that inside too.'
> ... 'But what for?'
> 'Control. To turn us into machines so we obey them,' Sybil whispered.'
>
> (Piercy 1976: 202)

These types of account all help to reinforce the feelings of powerlessness and lack of importance that fit the popular view of the mentally ill. It is especially borne out by narratives that see patients as objects for psychiatric professions to experiment upon as illustrated by the above extract or the following from Patrick McGrath's book *Asylum* concerning the doctor's view:

> Now that I had her here in the female wing I relished the prospect of stripping away her defences and opening her up, seeing what that psyche of hers really looked like. I understood of course that she would resist me but we had time.
>
> (McGrath 1996: 208)

It is clear that these examples only serve to build up the sense of scariness that the topic mental illness represents for both the sufferer and those around them. For the individual concerned there will be a fair amount of trepidation involved in seeking help or in disclosing their problems to others for fear of rejection or abuse. From the other perspective, the feeling of dangerousness posed by the mentally ill serves to reinforce and perpetuate the degree of distancing and exclusion subsequently encountered.

Making sense of literature

When reading a printed narrative, there are a number of factors which play a part in the final message that is taken away. First, we can look at the intention of the author as well as their ability to guide us towards a certain understanding that includes their narrative style and use of imagery and symbolism. Second, the readers themselves play a significant part in determining meaning by encoding a text in a specific way. The degree to which meaning is generated by a text is influenced to a large degree by the craft and intention of the author. As Sartre illustrates: 'The writer can guide you and, if he describes a hovel, make it seem the symbol of social injustice and provoke your indignation' (Sartre 1967: 3). This view states that it is the style of narrative which infuses life and depth to what is being related, guiding the reader towards the real significance of what is being recounted. It may also reflect Baudelaire's *double simultaneous postulation* where each word refers to two contexts, two forces being applied simultaneously to each phrase. Examples of this can be seen with allegorical narratives such as Joseph Heller's *Catch 22* or Franz Kafka's *Metamorphosis*. *Catch 22*, for example, can be read as a metaphorical account of madness, complete with its absurd logic and implied sense of impotence. The story *Metamorphosis* begins with the line: 'As Gregor Samsa awoke one morning from uneasy dreams he found himself transformed in his bed into a gigantic insect' (Kafka 1933: 9). It is a narrative that can also be read as a parable on human reaction to suffering and disease and the response of many towards mental illness. The significance of metaphorical and symbolic imagery is that the reader is required to suspend their rational thought and use their imagination in order to make sense of texts, thereby having new and provocative ways of exploring and understanding certain concepts and ideas.

Foucault (1979) questions the notion of the author being the presiding authority for the understanding of a text. This view reflects the concept of reception theory which states that a piece of writing cannot make sense independently but requires the intervention of an interpreting reader (Livingstone 1998; Holland 1980), which brings in the sense of collaboration between writer and reader, aptly illustrated by Sartre:

> On the one hand, the literary object has no substance but the reader's subjectivity . . . But on the other hand, the words are there like traps to arouse our feelings and to reflect them towards us . . . the work exists only at the exact level of his [the reader] capacities; while he reads and creates, he knows that he can always further in his reading, can always create more profoundly, and thus the work seems to him as inexhaustible . . . Thus the writer appeals to the reader's freedom to collaborate in the production of his work.
>
> (Sartre 1967: 31)

Readers hold a measure of power relating to the control of a story's flow, for example through reading a narrative in instalments (Armes 1994), as well as the understanding and comprehension they take away. This is illustrated by Young who asserts that: 'Meaning ... is not stable or fixed ... although authors may have intentions when they write, once they have written they cannot control and fix the meaning of any reading' (Young 1991: 238). This is borne out by the interpretative diversity brought by readers who have their own set of experiences and expectations from which to engage a particular text (Martin 1986). The notion of the interpretative reader limits the overall control that writers have as they can guide but they have no assurance as to what final meaning is taken away. It is an issue that can prove extremely frustrating for writers especially when their texts are misinterpreted, a fact bemoaned by Herman Hesse regarding his classic novel *Steppenwolf* (Hesse 2001). The role of the reader is highlighted by Bennett and Royle who illustrate two contrasting styles:

> Is reading simply something that happens to a text as if by chance, some-thing which leaves a text fundamentally unaltered? If so, then the role of reader would appear to be determined by the text itself: each literary text would be like a set of instructions, a kind of recipe for how it should be read. By contrast, the text may be understood as fundamentally incomplete, to be constructed in the act of reading. In this case the text is remade in every reading.
>
> (Bennett and Royle 1999: 16)

While some writing provides very clear guidance for the reader, other forms present a more open text with a plurality of potential interpretations (Barthes 1972). Opportunities are left for the reader to construct the meaning of a text and form their own interpretations. Another strand to consider is that of the reader undergoing changes between subsequent re-readings of a text, bring-ing with them a different mood and awareness of what happens next, resulting in an altered reading and a perceiving of new patterns (Martin 1986). We can see this process being influenced by a person's exposure to other media for-mats where new 'readings' or access to visual cues cause them to reinterpret what they know, for instance returning to Ken Kesey's *One Flew Over the Cuckoo's Nest* with an image of Jack Nicholson's charismatic screen char-acter in their minds. Another factor influencing a reader's engagement con-cerns their level of engagement with parts of a text either as an active or passive participant. It is a type of engagement that is not always constant and, as schema and script theories suggest, readers may alternate between the two. Augoustinos and Walker (1995) indicate that the existence of well-established representational knowledge structures favour a passive type of processing, in which the person does not perceive anything which contradicts their pre-conceptions and merely retraces former steps, reruns old experiences and treats the novel as familiar. Therefore, once a person has seen what they expect to see they may not challenge or question further. This reflects something of the mentally ill stereotype being accessed within a text without one really standing back and questioning the authenticity of the message being relayed. This concern can be matched by the uncertain degree of authority attached to many authors concerning the topic they are writing about. Having limited knowledge or insight into what one is writing was identified by Lothe (2000) as a major factor that makes a narrator unreliable. A brief look within the thriller and horror genres would appear to demonstrate that a large number of writers are unreliable sources when it comes to mental health content, opting for dramatic engagement of their readers over accurate portrayals.

The understanding that is taken away from works of literature is therefore subject to a variety of factors including both the intentions of the author as well as the particular interpretive framework applied by the reader. The importance from a health promotional point of view is to encourage further development of writing that presents mental illness from a better informed position as well as helping recipients to become more discerning and questioning about what they are reading.

Conclusion

The medium of literature has the ability to engage the reader more powerfully with the theme of mental illness than perhaps is achievable through other media sources. Of core significance here is the ability that this source has to engage the reader directly with the inner world (thoughts and feelings) of those involved, particularly through first-person narratives or autobiographical accounts. This medium provides a communication type that is rich in imagery, symbolism and narrative illustration, guiding those accessing it to construct their own pictures and understanding of the text before them. As has been illustrated above, the reader is provided with some very distinct associations concerning mental illness; on the one hand an all destructive process and on the other a survivable condition. The understanding about mental health issues gleaned from books is clearly to a large extent determined by the type of literary genre accessed. The dramatic potential that mental illness can bring to a text and its subsequent appeal for readers is perhaps too enticing for some authors to avoid. This means that the misleading, stereotypical and unrealistic forms of representation will continue to flourish. On a heartening note however, the increasingly popular reception of autobiographical accounts of distress is a welcome process in communicating more of the lived experience. Perhaps it should be noted that these predominantly feature mental health themes (i.e. abuse, eating disorders, alcoholism or surviving tragedy) that frame the person as *victim*, evoking feelings of sympathy and sorrow among their readers. It would be good to see this type of reception mirrored in other less-accepted mental health states such as schizophrenia, thereby helping the public to appreciate the reality of certain conditions more, and forming a base from which to challenge the many poorly-constructed representations accessible.

7 Film

The medium of film

For over a hundred years now viewers have been able to engage with the hugely appealing and attractive medium of film. Although not as popular today, at the beginning of the twentieth century moviegoers would queue in vast numbers to catch the latest releases. The cinema audience has progressively become more fragmented declining from 1,585 million in 1945 to 72 million in 1985 before rising to 140 million in 1999 (British Film Institute 2005). The overall fall in numbers is in part explained by increased competition from other developing media services, beginning perhaps with the advent of television in the 1950s and then the accessibility of film on video in the 1970s. In recent years the diversity of available products has widened further with cable and satellite services as well as new digital technology providing an almost overwhelming array of products to select from.

The medium of film has created a new channel for artistic and creative expression and has opened a new world of imagination by projecting the fantasies of writers and film-makers onto the screen (Bloom 1993). Prior to this, the mode of visual expression belonged predominantly to the world of art and the domain of stage production. Creative expression, utilising means such as drawing, painting or sculpture has for thousands of years been employed either as a means of recording and reporting or as a mode of stimulating and challenging creative thought. Hogarth's *Rake's Progress*, for example, documented the conditions and experiences of the mentally ill incarcerated within Bedlam hospital. Stage productions provided many features that were to later be captured and developed by the medium of film. Mood and atmosphere were first created by the presentation of the stage sets within which the drama took place. Against this background, the story was acted out using numerous visual and auditory modes of expression to enable audience members to engage with the overall set of messages being conveyed. It is a mode of storytelling that dates back over centuries, with a number of notable examples relaying mental illness themes to the audiences of their era. For example, the ancient Greek view of madness being manifested by the gods was reflected in a number of plays such as *The Bacchae* and *Heracles*.

There is also, of course, the important body of work produced by Shakespeare with numerous mental health references being found throughout his work in plays such as *King Lear* and *Macbeth*.

The innovation of reproductive imagery began at the beginning of the nineteenth century with developments of early photographic products such as the heliograph and the daguerreotype. This was matched by the creation of the moving image initially through various devices including the kineto-scope and the zoöpraxiscope but later, at the end of nineteenth century, with films by Thomas Eddison (*Fred Ott's Sneeze* 1894) and the Lumière brothers (*Workers Leaving the Lumière Factory* 1895). Sound recording initially pre-sented difficulties with regard to synchronisation, although found partial success through methods involving the tri-ergon process (a means of record-ing sound directly onto film), de Forest's phonofilm (using light as a method for writing and reading sound) and the vitaphone (a method of recording sound directly onto a disc). Clearly, these early initiatives seem primitive by comparison with modern film-making techniques but it is important to recognise how they might have been received by a fascinated public eager to enter more fully into the world created by the medium of film.

The ways in which we as an audience watch film is influenced by numer-ous lifestyle factors such as available time, cost issues and access to various technology and services. Films can be watched in the cinema as well as on television and computer screens, although it is in the cinema that viewers are presented with the most powerful engagement with the medium of film. This particular environment heightens the experience through reducing peri-pheral distracting stimuli and attracting the viewer more strongly towards what is presented before them. The reduction of external lighting and the large screen size means that our scope of vision is taken up exclusively with the film images projected before us. This is accompanied by a dominant volume of sound that helps to forcibly place us within the action being depicted. Our engagement with film is further influenced by audience mem-bers who share this experience with us and in a way act as guides towards particular emotional reactions that we might have in response to various scenes.

As Wedding and Boyd observe:

> When someone is watching a movie, an immediate bond is set up between the spectator and the film, and all the technical apparatus involved with the projection of the film becomes invisible as the images from the film pass into the spectator's consciousness. With the best films the viewer experiences a sort of dissociative state in which ordinary existence is temporarily suspended.
>
> (Wedding and Boyd 1999: 1)

The camera in a sense becomes what Metz (1982) refers to as our own viewing perspective as we collapse the distinction between our eyes and the projection apparatus. Unlike stage productions, the medium of film provides a more reliable means of ensuring that the viewer is looking where they ought to be looking (Carroll 1996). The importance of the visual stimuli engaged in by viewers is enhanced by the placing of a frame around it (Braudy 2002), and the methods used, including close-up shots and camera movement, are some of the many techniques used to guide an audience's attention and to provoke certain reactions. The final scene in Hitchcock's *Psycho*, for example, leads the viewer towards Norman Bates' eyes in order to draw them slowly and uncomfortably towards his disturbed and frightening world.

The medium of film engages audience members in various ways as Lothe states:

> Many film theorists have found that film, like music, works through atmosphere, resonance and rhythm. Film communication differs greatly from verbal language in that film is a language without a code and that understanding inferences etc. from a single camera shot may vary to the point of infinity.
>
> (Lothe 2000: 13)

The complexity of film as a communicating agent relates to the fact that it is much more than a set of observable cues, with a duality of sensory modes being employed. In essence, it covers the *auditory channel* (relating to noise, voice and music) as well as the *visual channel* that combines a range of camera and editing techniques (Chatham 1990). The issues outlined above highlight the intricacy of the messages being received through film and the multitude of stimuli to which we are exposed. As illustrated by Gestalt theory, film as an entire entity can be seen as being constructed from the intricate relationship of all its component parts. It is perhaps easier to understand the collective 'whole' by first exploring the various ways in which messages are transmitted. The depiction of mental health issues will be looked at with regard to imagery, narrative and sound (see Figure 7.1).

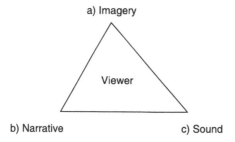

Figure 7.1 Film communication.

Film as a visual medium: imagery

As a visual medium, film provides a number of mental health representations that cover the whole spectrum from the sensitive and subtle through to the insensitive and grossly exaggerated. It is the latter type of depiction, though, that creates the greater impact and which is more memorable for the viewer. This can be reflected through the notion within perceptual theory of *figure and ground* whereby our attention is drawn towards a specific detail and, by focusing upon it, causes it to emerge from the background (King and Wertheimer 2005). Because film is not a static medium, the concept of what is figure and what is ground is constantly shifting as certain camera techniques cause our focus to move from one item to another. This then builds up a collective understanding as our glimpses of the background carry the context within which principal subjects are placed.

Characters/main subjects

Perhaps the first clue we are given regarding somebody's mental health state relates to the way in which they appear to us. The characterisation of mental illness is usually achieved through various stereotypical cues that leave the audience with little difficulty in discriminating between those who have mental health problems and those who do not. Wahl (1995) refers to this as the portrayal of the mentally ill as '*a breed apart*', made different by virtue of their looks and behaviour. One of the more deliberate ways of presenting mental illness is through the casting of actors who look odd or different. A notable example of this was the selection of Peter Lorre who played a series of 'mad' and deranged characters. His build, facial features, large eyes and 'creepy' Eastern European accent provided film-makers with what has been described as a textbook illustration of schizophrenia (Wahl 1995). Another example of intentionally casting people who look 'mad' can be seen in the film *One Flew over the Cuckoo's Nest* where some actors were selected because their appearance fitted stereotypical notions of the mentally ill. One choice in particular was the casting of Michael Berryman as the tall bald patient. He was already a 1970s horror genre icon because of his distinctive features, a rare medical condition resulting in him having no hair, fingernails or teeth. A counter perhaps to the many typically unattractive characterisations of the mentally ill is provided by a variety of more engaging and charismatic ones such as Jack Nicholson as the obsessive compulsive Melvin Udall in the film *As Good As It Gets*, Russell Crowe as John Nash in *A Beautiful Mind* and Judy Dench as Iris Murdoch in the film *Iris*. A further issue linked with characterisation relates to the presence of accompanying cues that serve to provide clues as to a person's mental health state, highlighting certain features such as dangerousness. The excessive use of restraint devices for Hannibal Lecter in the film *The Silence of the Lambs* and Freddy Krueger's (*Nightmare on Elm Street*) cadaverous look and bladed gloves all help to exacerbate the sense of threat posed.

Background

There are a number of the ways in which mood or complementary under-standing is created by virtue of the background within which scenes are enacted upon. In some cases, the exterior setting acts almost as a mirror, providing the viewer with a visual enactment of specific characteristics or elements being covered. This is observed by Bobker (1969) in relation to the film *Through a Glass Darkly* where the character of the sunlight (flat, grey and totally lacking in warmth) can be seen as an external projection of the internal conflicts and hopelessness felt with regard to the daughter's schizo-phrenia. Another example can be seen in the film *One Flew over the Cuckoo's Nest* where the dull, colourless and impersonal background perfectly reflects the overall climate of care. It is also interesting to note the way in which the chaotic world of madness is depicted in the artistic, stage-type sets employed in the silent German film *The Cabinet of Dr Caligari*. This is helped by the angular, asymmetrical and unfinished aspect of the scenery that serves to unsettle and disorient the viewer.

Film as an auditory medium: narrative and sound

Narrative

The style of narrative found within films reflects something of the prevailing attitudes towards the topic of mental illness. It is at times sensitive, thought-ful and funny and at other times offensive, cruel and uninformed. To some degree it relates to the film as a whole and the type of reaction that film-makers are trying to evoke in their audience. The impact that specific words have is not solely down to what is said but also relates strongly to the context within which they appear. For example, the film *One Flew over the Cuckoo's Nest* includes a number of seemingly derogatory and stigmatising statements including McMurphy's: 'We're nuts, we're in the mental defectives league.' However, the prevailing attitude from McMurphy towards his fellow patients is respectful and caring and the words used come across less as insults and more as self-parody. This can also be reflected in some of the language in the film *Arsenic and old Lace* concerning the highly 'eccentric' Brewster family: 'Madness doesn't run in our family it gallops.' While these examples are more of the benevolent kind, the same cannot be said of *Me, Myself and Irene* and the use of terms such as 'You've got a screw loose', 'psycho' and 'schizo'. This film also displays a marked change in vocal style between the split person-alities of Hank and Charlie, with Hank, for example, adopting a menacing Clint Eastwood style drawl. These references are unashamedly used with little consideration being shown for the offence they might cause. Fortunately there are films that provide examples of a softer and more caring dialogue as shown by Suzanna's (*Girl Interrupted*) statement: 'Crazy isn't being broken, it's just me and you amplified.' The range of examples therefore found within the medium of film is very mixed and deciding whether they are positive or negative depends upon the 'global' characterisation of mental illness being depicted.

Sound

The purpose of film music is reflected in the broad functions outlined by Prendergast (1992); these include:

- Creating atmosphere
- Underlining the psychological states of characters
- Providing neutral background fillers
- Building a sense of continuity
- Sustaining tension and then rounding it off with a sense of closure

As illustrated by these characteristics, film scores are evocative of mood and music can generate feeling, be it peacefulness and tranquillity or imminent danger. As Devereaux and Hillman state: 'Music can seek to represent in sound a written text' (Devereaux and Hillman 1995:183). As an example, they cite Hitchcock's 1943 film *Shadow of a Doubt* and the choice of the Merry Widow waltz (a piece of music embellished with horror harmonies) for a story concerning a homicidal maniac with a penchant for widows. In another film, *Through a Glass Darkly*, there is a sense of fragmentation between the film scenes and music which do not quite synchronise, both being allowed in a sense to go their own way. This, according to Bobker (1969), accompanied by the bleak, dark character of Bach's Cello Suite number 2, reveals something of the daughter's schizophrenic world.

Sound and music act as a powerful communicator telling us, for instance, when a significant moment is happening and indicating what we should feel about it (Turner 1999). This is supported by Frith who states: 'Music amplifies the mood or atmosphere and also tries to convey the emotional significance of a scene' (Frith 1986: 65). A notable example here is Hitchcock's shower scene from *Psycho* where the sense of danger and suspense are power-fully evoked through the unnerving and shrieking violin strings that appear cruel, painful and murderous when matched with the descending knife (Carroll 1996). There is also the significance of certain screen characters having their own signature tune, or *leitmotif*, when a particular recurring style of music is played in order to help characterise a person.

Lastly, when considering the importance of sound it is worth reflecting upon its absence and the deliberate use of silence. As has been addressed above, a disturbing and frightening feeling can be evoked in the audience member by the use of loud music, fragmented orchestration and screeching violin strings. An equally disturbing mood can be created by removing sound or reducing volume, thereby leaving viewers with either a confused auditory experience or a feeling of agonising suspense. The film *Psycho* provides a vivid example of this where immediately preceding the detective's murder, the volume is reduced to a very quiet state in order to unsettle and discomfort the viewer who is thereby alerted in a different way to what is expected (music becoming louder) and to the imminent presence of danger.

The sender

While the text of a novel can be regarded as a complete entity in itself, the scriptwriter provides a text that is designed to serve as a stimulus to the actors who, under the guidance of a director, offer a personal interpretation of each character (Armes 1994). The performance, therefore, that reaches the spectator is not purely the version offered by the scriptwriter but one that contains interpretations and influences from a number of others. It is also subject to change owing to related regulations and issues of censorship. A point made by the British Film Institute (2005) is that the moving image is subject to far greater censorship than any other artistic medium, with film and video releases in Britain being among the most tightly regulated in the Western world. Indeed, there are a variety of legislative and regulatory processes governing the medium of film, the first piece of British legislation being the Cinematograph Act (1909) which provided for the licensing of exhibition premises and the safety of audiences. This was followed by a number of cinematograph acts before these were all eventually replaced by the 1985 Films Act. A further piece of legislation relating to the release of film on video was provided by the Video Recordings Act (1984) which was set up to control and restrict the amount of obscene material, sex and violence included. The focus on screen content has been reflected in a number of acts covering a range of subjects including cruelty to animals (Cinematograph Films (Animals) Act 1937), obscenity (Obscene Publications Act 1959 – extended to cover films in 1977), indecent images of children (Protection of Children Act 1978), freedom of expression (Human Rights Act 1998), as well as various types of criminal activity (Criminal Justice Act 1994).

Two major organisations concerned with film classification are the aptly named British Board of Film Classification (BBFC) (formerly British Board of Film Censors), and the Motion Picture Association of America (MPAA). Neither of these organisations has any legal status with regard to film censorship but they carry out their regulatory role in collaboration with local authorities. The local authorities hold the main power and may decide to ignore the board's decisions as, for example, with the banning of the films *A Clockwork Orange* and *Crash* despite their gaining BBFC approval. Both the BBFC and MPAA provide ratings as to who watches what although there is little direct reference made to mental health themes. The BBFC provide classification relating to the themes of:

- Language
- Nudity

- Sex
- Violence
- Imitable techniques
- Horror
- Drugs

The MPAA covers similar themes and it is surprising to note that besides drug abuse and aspects concerning suicide and self-harm, no direct reference is made to mental health content. This appears to be an ongoing problem dating back to the earliest days of film regulation. Indeed, the British Board of Film Censors covered 43 aspects within their 1913–1915 annual report as satisfying grounds for deletion, covering nothing about disability or mental health issues besides a single reference to 'The drug habit'. The theme of drug addiction is one that causes considerable concern and one that was listed as the most concerning topic by the public in a BBFC (2005) report. An example from the United States relates to the 1955 film about drug addiction, *The Man with the Golden Arm*. This was initially banned by the Maryland State Board of Censors but later released by the Court of Appeals with the ruling that the film did not advocate the use of narcotics and was likely to act as a deterrent. However, a 30-second scene showing Frank Sinatra preparing heroin in a spoon was required to be deleted (Grazia and Newman 1982). Within the British Board Film of Classification (2000) publication *Sense and Sensibilities: Public Opinion & the BBFC Guidelines*, a small majority (52 per cent) agreed that films should be allowed to portray drug use in a realistic manner although there were mixed views regarding the portrayal of method. Calls have been made for film-makers to demonstrate a social responsibility in the messages and themes they are portraying with anti-drug portrayals being regarded as preferable to pro-drug ones (Valenti 2000). It is a point that could be debated with regard to the receipt of film content by different audience members using as illustration the film *Trainspotting* which could be viewed either as a glamorisation of drug culture or as a powerful anti-drug message.

Despite there being few references made concerning the portrayal of mental health content it is perhaps surprising to note that in 1928 the BBFC wanted to ban Robert Wiene's *Cabinet of Dr Caligari*, afraid that the asylum scenes might upset people in the cinema audience who had relatives in mental health hospitals (Film Education 2005). Other films with mental health content that have met with the BBFC's disapproval include Roman Polanski's *Repulsion* and Samuel Fuller's *Shock Corridor*. The BBFC's consultant, Dr Stephen Black, expressed concerns about *Repulsion*'s fantasy rape scenes (shown as part of Catherine Deneuve's delusional and paranoid mental state) although the film was passed uncut. *Shock Corridor* however was banned in 1963 for suggesting that residency in a mental hospital could induce insanity. The BBFC refused to grant a certificate saying that depiction of conditions in an American mental asylum bore no comparison with hospitals in Britain. It was also stated that the film might frighten cinemagoers who had relatives in mental institutions (Mathews 1994). This is an interesting response although the emergent views about the detrimental effects of long-term institutional care expressed by Goffman (1961), Barton (1976) and Scheff (1974) are per-haps far more alarming than the images depicted in film. What is not lost, though, is the degree of sensitivity and concern being demonstrated by the BBFC in these instances concerning the potential negative impact of mental health themes being depicted. However the laudability of this type of response is let down by the overall level of inconsistency shown as many other misleading and sometimes appalling examples, such as *Me, Myself and Irene*, are passed unchallenged. There has long been a culture of depicting the disabled and mentally ill in a negative and unproductive light and such destructively stigmatising messages can in the long term prove exceedingly damaging to those with mental health problems and their families. What is required is a much more direct focus being applied within the regulatory guidelines concerning the topic of mental illness.

The historical picture

Film has been described by some as a mirror, whereby the images of insanity presented bear a unique relationship with fluctuations in psychological theory and practice (Flemming and Manvell 1994). The extent to which cinematic images either reflect societal attitudes or in some cases create them is open to debate. Certainly, there are some very powerful and impactful film depictions that still resonate many years after their first screening. The film *Psycho*, for instance, has left us with a negative term of reference and association that is still very much in evidence within everyday speech and newspaper headlines (Welch and Racine 1999).

Starting with early cinematic releases at the beginning of the twentieth century we can see examples such as *The Escaped Lunatic* (1904), *Dr Dippy's Sanitarium* (1906), or even the Stan Laurel film *Nuts in May* (1917). The titles alone present a very disparaging and ridiculing view creating the feeling that 'mad' people belong in institutions. This was an era when the population of institutions was on the increase, maintaining the largely held view that incarcer-ation was beneficial both to society as well as the mentally ill. These early portrayals depicted the mentally ill either as monsters or as comically insane seemingly little bothered about the feelings or experiences of those concerned.

The 1930s and 1940s provided a contrast to the preceding era with a degree of ridicule extending towards those treating mental illness and the portrayals were often of comic figures treating sane individuals. In the 1940s and 1950s Hollywood turned its attention to the social problem film (e.g. *The Man with the Golden Arm* and drug addiction) covering many different issues and including themes relating to mental illness (Gabbard and Gabbard 1999). The late 1950s and early 1960s could be seen as the 'Golden Age' with an idealised view of psychiatry being represented. It reflected the growing conviction that psychiatrists were the authoritative voices of reason, adjustment and well-being. It was also interestingly an era that heralded the introduction of a major new product within the domain of mental health care, namely pheno-thiazine medication, thus further strengthening the power and authority afforded the medical practitioner. The mid- to late 1960s and the 1970s was denoted by Gabbard and Gabbard (1999) as the 'Fall from Grace', corresponding with a growing disillusionment with psychiatric care as the detrimental effects of institutional care became more apparent. These aspects are clearly outlined in a number of films including Milos Forman's *One Flew over the Cuckoo's Nest* and Mark Robson's *Bedlam*.

The shift towards community care and the enhanced visibility of mental health problems in society has culminated in the growing trend of showing the viewer more of an individual's felt experience of mental health problems. Films such as *A Beautiful Mind* and *Iris* present us with characters with whom viewers can readily form an emotional attachment, feeling compassion and sorrow for their sense of loss and experience of fragmenting worlds. It is a welcome change from other contemporary films that perpetuate stereo-typical notions of the mentally ill as violent (Hannibal Lecter series) or schizophrenia as a split personality (*Me, Myself and Irene*).

The message

This section addresses two core themes, that of the cinematic depiction of mental illness as well as the portrayal of treatment. The ways in which mental illness is depicted within the medium of film can be viewed via a number of different categories. For the purposes of this book the chosen areas are *the mentally ill* as the killer, the afflicted genius and the comic/eccentric. These are adapted from the themes portrayed in Radio 4's *Back Row* programme (4th May 2002) concerning the portrayal of mental illness and learning disabilities in the cinema.

The killer

Cinematic history contains countless examples of portraying the mentally ill as killers. There is an extra chilling edge added to the mentally ill killer as a consequence of their uncertain state of mind, and they are often shown as being deranged, frenzied or detached. It seems that over the decades, sub-sequent films each go a stage further in dispatching their victims in an ever more grisly fashion, with increased carnage and ferocity being depicted. These characters range in presentations from those whose altered psycho-logical state is merely seen as a transient phase to others who are deemed hopelessly insane and who will never recover, for example the psychopathic killer Michael Myers in the film *Halloween*.

The continued association between violence and mental illness is one that is heavily influenced by its popularity as well as the enhanced level of excitement or drama it adds. Many of these types of film attract large audiences and sometimes even critical acclaim, responses that help to ensure their continued appearance (Wahl 1995). The ongoing success of 'slasher' films perhaps relates to a societal desire for 'monsters' and the cathartic needs which are met through watching certain films. This is highlighted by Wolfenstein and Leites who state that: 'It is a perennial function of drama and literature to present images of what violent impulses, usually restrained in life, might look like if more fully expressed' (Wolfenstein and Leites 1970: 175). We are thus able to quench our curiosity and confront the 'monsters' that lurk in society while in what is perceived to be a safe and contained environment. At the end of the film we can leave the cinema or switch off the television and return to a feeling of secure normality. A problem with this is that some of these disturbing images and associations remain with us. As demonstrated through the process of classical conditioning and the reinforcement of associated stimuli (Pavlov 1958), the continued link between mental health problems and violence only serve to perpetuate the dangerousness myth. As Byrne (2001a) states, many films reinforce two misconceptions, mental illness as violence and the belief that every mentally ill person harbours one 'great dark secret'. Despite all the educative messages to the contrary that the general public are exposed to, this continued association leaves the viewer with a general feeling of unease. One consequence of this is a desire of some to place distance (physically and psychologically) between themselves and those with mental health problems. It is not surprising therefore to hear of the opposition by certain local communities towards plans for the placing of those with mental health problems within their midst, with the misassumption that they pose a significant threat of danger.

A number of grossly misrepresented facts permeate our collective body of knowledge and become integrated to a large extent within our culture and language. This is illustrated by Welch and Racine (1999) who point out that the term 'psycho' has become a byword for terrifying, homicidal impulses, or the unpredictability of a deranged mind. Cinema creates a number of lasting and dramatic impressions that are readily accepted by those who wish to add extra spice to reported events as shown in the newspaper headline '*Silence of the Lambs* Maniac Freed to Kill' (*Today*). It seems that the power of these images is such that they extend beyond the confines of their original film. The stereotypical killer may be ridiculous, farcical and totally exaggerated although some such as Hannibal Lecter and Freddy Krueger have managed to achieve a wide degree of popularity, even a type of cult hero status.

It is interesting to note the variation in type of character selected to represent the mentally deranged killer and their relationship to the victims. Two broad types of representation include the murderer as somebody known to the victim and someone who is not. The first category features the unsettling representation of the killer who is already in our midst. It is the individual who is trusted and liked and perhaps the least suspected by their unfortunate victim. It may be a friend ('Good old Bob' – the serial killer in *Frenzy*); the family man who goes berserk (as with Jack Nicholson in *The Shining*), or even a trusted health care professional (the cannibalistic and nightmarish Hannibal Lecter in *The Silence of the Lambs* or Michael Caine as the murderous transvestite in *Dressed to Kill*). The impact of these types of portrayal is the sense that no matter how rational or well-presented those with mental health problems seem, there is a feeling they may perhaps be a 'ticking time bomb', slowly winding up towards their murderous and frenzied explosion. This illustrates the insidious nature of stigmatisation whereby certain views and connections are strongly held irrespective of any messages that are presented to the contrary. It highlights the feeling of unsettlement and mistrust which can be attached to those who are unfortunate enough to be labelled mentally ill, even family members and friends who, pre-diagnosis, were regarded in a wholly different light.

The second type of categorisation signifies the threat posed should our safe and secure world come into contact, however chance or random, with those who are mentally unstable. This meeting however fleeting is portrayed in a number of films (e.g. *Enduring Love, Play Misty for Me* or *Fatal Attraction*) as having murderous consequences. Other films depict the random slaying of whoever happens, unluckily, to be in the wrong place at the wrong time. These killers often use excessive savagery and ferocity in the dispatch of their hapless victims such as that seen in *Natural Born Killers* or *The Texas Chainsaw Massacre*. Despite educative messages to the contrary, such as that provided by the Department of Health's (1999) Safer Services report, the desire for security and safety leaves a number of individuals desiring a sense of distance from the mentally ill.

Afflicted genius

This is a fascinating category as it engages strong sympathetic feelings and affords opportunities to get closer to the individual concerned. To a large extent it depends upon the way in which they are portrayed as, on one side of the spectrum, we have the deranged, power-mad individuals, whereas, on the other, are the struggling genius types hampered by their mental health state. The former group are shown as obsessively driven towards their goal, be it the creation of life (*Frankenstein, The Island of Dr Moreau*) or the striving for power (as for instance with most of the James Bond villains). The more sensitive portrayal centres on the talented individual who has become handicapped by their fragmenting state of mind. The feeling evoked in the audience might be one of pity for their plight or a real sense of loss for their declining abilities. The core theme here is of the central figure striving to cope with their affliction. A number of recent films have created a sense of attraction by focusing upon 'based upon a true story' scripts and by choosing charismatic and popular actors to play the main parts. All of these aspects help to create a real sense of emotional connectedness in the viewer and a liking for the main characters. The '*real story*' theme means that their talent is not simply imagined and is an approach that stirs stronger feelings of sympathy within their audience. For example, in the film *Iris* we follow the writer Iris Murdoch on her painfully distressing journey as she loses what is most important to her and her prodigious talent: words. One scene painfully depicts Iris struggling through a cognitive assessment, unable to name even the simplest of items such as a spoon or a tennis racquet. It is a heartbreaking and tragic process to witness, and reflects a process that is also played out in other films featuring gifted individuals as seen with the brilliant mathematician John Nash (*A Beautiful Mind*).

From a cynical point of view these films might be criticised for their lack of realism regarding the ordinary person who is most represented within mental health problem statistics. Taking a different stance we might consider Landesman's remark regarding the disability film *The Sea Inside* that: 'Somewhere in the world there must be a disabled person who is boring. Someone who has no talent for writing, maths or science; who is not brave and witty, but has bad breath and cracks terrible jokes' (Landesman 2005: 19). Obviously this could also refer to the mentally ill, many of whom do not possess a remarkable talent. The focus upon genius or gifted ability, while helping to distance a film from the many made-for-television 'true life stories', is perhaps the prime factor being offered in terms of providing the audience with a vehicle for acceptance. These individuals' special talents transgress their fragile mental health states and allow them as a consequence to be better accommodated by the audience. A scene in the film *Shine* gives a very vivid example of this as the shabby and dishevelled David Helfgott shuffles into a posh bar and moves through an unsettled crowd towards the piano. The jeering calls do not deter him and a few chords into his playing of Rachmaninov's *Third Piano Concerto* brings about an almost hushed reverence. His outstanding performance is greeted with loud applause and he is promptly installed as their resident pianist, all previous doubts about him apparently dismissed. In a sense his talented genius transforms and reclassifies his mentally ill status into that of the more tolerable and accepted one of 'eccentric'. It reflects the criticism levelled at this film that: 'If mentally ill, you can only make it in society, or are acceptable if you are a genius, or famous or on the path to fame' (Rosen and Walter 2000: 239). Likewise, John Nash (*A Beautiful Mind*), because of his prodigious mathematics talent, is accommodated and accepted by many on campus despite his increasingly bizarre and erratic behaviour.

There is obviously a gulf between the experience of mental illness depicted in these types of films and the reality felt by many so-called 'ordinary' people. The showcasing of a talented individual provides the audience member perhaps with an added level of appeal. This is complemented by the intriguing and compelling focus upon that person's fragmented mental health state. It is an issue raised by Rosen and Walter (2000) who state that if you are mentally ill, and talented, the audience will only take an interest if they can gawk voyeuristically at your bizarre antics, no matter how interested they are in your talent. This statement illustrates further the attractiveness of this dramatic subject matter to both film-makers and audience members and reflects one of the prime reasons why a person's illness is given so much prominence over other aspects of their life which are largely ignored.

Despite the problems inherent in this type of film, there is a valuable opportunity afforded to establish a degree of understanding regarding the lived experience of mental health problems. The biographical focus enables us as viewers to follow the person showcased and develop an interest and even a feeling of caring about their life. John Nash's desperate struggles, for example, convey the serious impact his mental health state has on his ability to function and the distressing consequences for his family. The close relationship formed between audience member and principal character means that the viewer will have specific feelings aroused by the events unfolding before them on the screen. It might involve an appreciation of the sense of fear and frustration felt or simply an understanding of the alienation and rejection experienced by many of those encountering mental health problems and their families.

Comic/eccentric

It is evident that in most instances within the comic/eccentric categorisation the principal focus is upon entertaining the audience to the detriment of actually highlighting the reality of the experience being portrayed. Perhaps one of the crucial factors relating to the comedic portrayal of mental illness concerns the audience's engagement with characters and whether they are laughing with them or at them. On the negative side, viewers are provided with opportunities to be amused and entertained by the bizarre and 'clownish' antics of the mentally ill with many stereotypes being employed. These depictions generally present characters for the audience to laugh *at*, an approach that does not foster feelings of concern for their welfare. On the positive side, there are some engaging portrayals featuring characters who are on the whole liked by the audience. A core difference here relates to the enticement of the audience to laugh *with* screen characters, in a number of instances recognising aspects familiar in their own lives.

One type of depiction in this category is of the harmless eccentric, something in sharp contrast to that of the 'mentally ill as killer' classification. Two vivid examples of this can be seen with James Stewart as Elwood P. Dowd, the jovial and hallucinating alcoholic (*Harvey*), and Uncle Teddy, who believes he is Teddy Roosevelt (*Arsenic and Old Lace*). The characters illustrated here are not people to be scared of, as with the 'killer' category, but rather to be pitied, tolerated or amused by. The pursuit of incarceration for each of the examples raised here are less about removing them for the protection of others but seem to be more generated by feelings of benevolence. Both Elwood and Teddy are reasonably well tolerated and accepted by their families despite their fairly unusual behaviours. Elwood has an imaginary friend, a large white rabbit named Harvey, whom only he can see, whereas Teddy believes he is the president of the United States and is busy building the Panama Canal in his basement. The insistence that Teddy is 'unwell' and will be 'happy at Happydale' seems more farcical because it appears as if the entire Brewster family is in need of help. The film *Arsenic and Old Lace* provides an interesting collection of representations of madness with both the comic killer and the harmless eccentric being portrayed alongside each other. As well as the aforementioned Uncle Teddy, Cary Grant puts in an exhaustively manic performance as Mortimer Brewster, another apparently harmless eccentric. On the other hand, the comedic killer is depicted by the surgically disfigured brother Jonathan, a murderer on the run with his plastic surgeon sidekick (played by Peter Lorre), as well as Aunts Abby and Martha who have been poisoning gentleman visitors and burying them in the cellar. It is perhaps made more ludicrous with the singling out of Teddy, on whom the family's madness is projected, as the sole person in need of treatment. This wonderfully illustrates the process of displacement as seen with the old asylum culture whereby certain individuals were designated as mentally ill and removed from their families for treatment.

The comedic representation is not always a benign one as it also offers up offensive characterisations or portrayals that evoke a sense of ridicule and disparagement. It is here that the entertainment needs of the audience are placed securely before any considerations being shown concerning the mentally ill. A prime example of this is the film *Me, Myself and Irene* which shows the character played by Jim Carrey struggling between his distinct states of wellness and illness. There are many classic stereotypes being played out here including those of the depiction of schizophrenia as a split personality. Charlie represents the mentally well state and is a caring although submissive person, whereas Hank, the mentally ill one, is loud, abrasive and abusive. It is a film that has been largely criticised by mental health groups such as Mind (2000) for its harmful reinforcement of a number of stereotypes concerning mental illness. This film differs significantly from those illustrated above in that there is nothing likeable about Jim Carrey's Hank. While the audience might laugh at the absurdity of the scenes being relayed, it is actually a disturbing and deeply offensive portrayal that does much to harm society's developing attitudes and awareness towards the mentally ill.

A further aspect engaging the audience in a laughing *with* response concerns the depiction of the neurotic. This representation is perhaps the closest and most easily identifiable representation for many audience members. It presents a form less associated with severe psychiatric disturbance and something more aligned to the quirkiness of individual characters. To a large extent those centred upon are likeable characters with their neuroses providing the audience with moments for amusement as well as sympathetic concern. A prime example here can be seen with the angst ridden character played by Woody Allen in a number of his films such as *Annie Hall* and *Play it Again Sam*. Another good example is reflected by the ridiculous sense of incongruity provided by the film *Analyze This* as the neurotic mobster boss (Robert

DeNiro) seeks treatment for anxiety. It presents a stark contrast when compared with the usual screen portrayal of a mobster as fearless and ruthless. What is interesting about many of the neurotic representations is the sense of connectedness fostered with the audience member. As with Woody Allen's agitated mannerisms and ceaseless pacing before landing a date in the film *Annie Hall*, it is perhaps easy for many to identify with the excruciating intensity felt when asking somebody out on a first date. Although the intensity of experience might be different to that being depicted on the screen, the audience are still offered a number of points of engagement whereby difficulties and problems shown are understood.

Audience response

The categories listed above of killer, afflicted genius and comic/eccentric all lead the viewer towards a distinctly different way of relating to the mentally ill. First, we can regard the depiction of the psychopathic killer as leading the viewer towards a position of fear and unsettlement. Second, the categorisation of afflicted genius serves to engage pitying and sympathetic reactions. This is mainly evoked by highlighting a person's plight and the sense of the tragedy regarding what they have lost or are consequently unable to do. The third categorisation of comic/eccentric engenders feelings of amusement through laughing directly *at* characters or *with* them. The implications here for learning about mental health issues are to a large degree dependent upon the type of characterisations that individuals are exposed to as each has the capacity to evoke very different feelings and attitudes. Individuals will therefore be drawn towards certain responses and understanding by virtue of which genres they select for viewing although further reinforcers will also be obtained from other media sources that individuals are exposed to. Particular characterisations such as 'the killer' could be regarded as having a greater influence than the others because of the fear factor involved and the general absence of likeable traits. This is to some degree countered by the latter two groups which on the whole include the more likeable and identifiable representations, more of which are certainly needed.

Mental health treatment

Cinematic history contains a wide array of examples demonstrating mental health treatment and the individuals who offer it. There is on the whole an overrepresentation of talking cures and hypnosis within films and an under-representation of pharmacotherapy or medical approaches such as electro-convulsive therapy (ECT), unless included for dramatic social control effects or as a form of punishment. These depictions appear polarised and from the earliest days of cinema, films either idealised or degraded the mental health profession (Greenberg and Gabbard 1990). This may vary from the sense of awe and omnipotence afforded to psychiatrists in their so-called golden era (Gabbard and Gabbard 1999) to a general discreditation through the serving up of harsh, uncaring and controlling approaches. It is a view supported by Clare who states that: 'Psychiatrists as seen through the eyes of filmmakers are at one and the same time omnipotent and useless, progressive and reactionary, compassionate and destructive, perceptive and blind' (Clare 2001: ch. 2, sec. 4). Alternatively, this variation can be summed up in the categories identified by Schneider (1987) of Dr Dippy, Dr Evil and Dr Wonderful. A further issue concerns the confusion as to the background of those who are actually providing care because of the tendency to merge together the different professions portrayed (Tam 2002). This point is further highlighted by Gabbard and Gabbard (1992) who state that Hollywood portrayals often do not distinguish between psychiatrists, psychoanalysts and psychologists.

The confusing plethora of messages found within the medium of film reflects that presented by other media providers. The type of material exposed to and the way in which it is portrayed will no doubt influence expectations and feelings about treatment. As indicated by Gabbard and Gabbard: 'Psychiatric patients come to the consulting room with expectations of how a psychiatrist should behave based on what they see in the movies' (Gabbard and Gabbard 1999: 177). Dependent therefore on which films have been seen, individuals will have very different feelings about mental health treatment. This is demonstrated by the extreme range of examples on offer as there are, for instance, the oppressive and regimented care as depicted in *One Flew Over The Cuckoo's Nest*, the paternalistic asylum approach in *Quills*, the comic/ ineffective approach in *The Couch Trip*, the sensitive, tireless and determined help in *Awakenings* and the murderous, psychopathic approach in *The Silence of the Lambs* or *Dressed to Kill*. The impact that film can have upon attitudes towards mental illness was illustrated by Domino's (1983) study concerning the film *One Flew over the Cuckoo's Nest* that observed a less positive attitude being demonstrated by those who had seen the film. Although this study was questioned by Secker and Platt (1996) because of what they identified as research design weaknesses it nonetheless raises some very important questions concerning the potential impact of film upon resultant attitudes. This is illustrated by Tim Lott in his autobiographical work *A Scent of Dried Roses* where he states that: 'The idea of tablets and treatments remains beyond the pale; they [his parents] too have seen *One Flew over the Cuckoo's Nest*' (Lott 1997: 238). It is easy therefore to understand the extra sense of trepidation felt when seeking care or even avoiding it altogether given the depersonalising and brutal treatment regime portrayed very powerfully in this particular film.

The positive side of care is illustrated by appealing role models like the psychologist Sean Maguire (Robin Williams) in *Good Will Hunting* or Dr Berger (Judd Hirsch) in the film *Ordinary People*. They provide us with a glimpse of the sort of carer we would perhaps hope to encounter if we were feeling vulnerable and in need of support as both of them present as

jargon-free, approachable, caring and unpretentious. Films containing positive and caring role models who are properly able to connect with those they
are treating stand as a positive advertisement for mental health care. They
also help to challenge the wealth of negative examples accessible and are
encouraging for those who are uncertain about seeking help. While presenting us with a very desirous image of carers who actually do seem to care,
potential problems may be caused for individuals whose own experience falls
short of any subsequently held expectations. This is especially illustrated by
Clare's (2001) observation that positive role models tend towards idealised
interpretations and include the common portrayal of psychoanalysts as an
amalgam between Sherlock Holmes and Sigmund Freud. Another unrealistic
representation is the tireless activist who is prepared to risk all in the interests
of their patients, a portrayal strongly conveyed in the film *Awakenings*. It
follows the familiar tradition of the police action film depicting the hero
improbably risking his badge and his life in the pursuit of justice. The
image of the idealised carer is contrasted by a number of examples portraying
them in a far from perfect light. As Gabbard (2001) indicates, the denigration
of psychiatrists neutralises something of their perceived omniscience and
shows they have the same human frailties as everyone else. This can be seen in
a number of films such as *High Anxiety* or *The Couch Trip* where it becomes
questionable as to who is most in need of therapy, those giving it or those
receiving it.

The screen image can be extremely evocative and engaging as shown in the
final cathartic breakthrough and tearful hug with Dr Berger in *Ordinary
People* where the guilt held over Conrad's brother's death is finally laid to
rest. The cathartic breakthrough is usually included in scenes towards the end
of films and is the culmination of a difficult and at times fraught process. A
criticism that could be levelled at such scenes involves the over-dramatisation
of the therapeutic process and the presentation of a number of inaccuracies.
Such misrepresentations not only prove confusing for those receiving care but
can also lead to therapists encouraging cathartic interventions when it is not
what the client has come for (Jinks 2000). Another common cinematic portrayal is the sudden recovery of repressed memories, an aspect recognised by
Freud as in itself not being curative. As Gabbard and Gabbard state: 'If
filmmakers have studied the history of the psychoanalytic movement, it would
seem that they stopped reading Freud's work at this particular historical
point' (Gabbard and Gabbard 1999: 28). It seems therefore that film-makers
are more concerned with enticing and engaging their viewers with dramatic
scenes than in presenting accuracy. This is particularly illustrated by *The
Three Faces of Eve* (1957), where it remains a mystery for viewers as to how
finally remembering childhood trauma actually cures her illness.

Although it is heartening to note the number of films depicting mental
health care in a positive light they are perhaps outnumbered by those carrying
a negative message. Physical treatments in particular are much maligned providing the film-maker with opportunities for visually dramatic scenes. One

such method is ECT which, although initially shown in films such as the 1948 film *The Snake Pit* as a severe but helpful remedy for personal distress, has become progressively portrayed as a more negative and cruel treatment, leaving the impression of a brutal and abusive treatment that has little therapeutic benefit (McDonald and Walter 2001; Hodgkinson 1986). This is evidenced within the film *One Flew over the Cuckoo's Nest* where a crowd of people await McMurphy as he enters the treatment room suggesting to the viewer that there is no room for refusal. The scene in itself makes this particular treatment method appear cruel and uncaring, more concerned with issues of social control than of benevolent care. The themes of control and punishment are strongly reinforced throughout this film ending with McMurphy being lobotomised as a final attempt to control his 'disruptive' behaviour. The problem with such powerfully negative stereotypes of care is that it may lead those seeking or receiving mental health care to expect that they will somehow also be violated or abused (Gabbard and Gabbard 1999). Even though individuals are also exposed to other sources of information, examples such as these convey very powerful messages that can be hard to overcome.

Lastly, it is worth mentioning here a popular theme among film-makers, that of an individual recovering through the power of love (Byrne 2001b). It is a theme occurring in numerous films such as *Crazy People, As Good As It Gets* and *Shine* providing salvation for an individual who is struggling with issues of mental distress. The suggestion that love can be sufficiently powerful to overcome one's psychological difficulties could in some instances be regarded as trivialising the serious nature of mental illness. It does however help to stress a crucial component of the therapeutic relationship that relates to the Rogerian concept of feeling connected with and cared for (Rogers 1961). It also reflects the recognition that feelings of separation, disconnectedness and isolation have a significant impact upon one's mental well-being (Maslow 1971; Kitwood 1997; Social Exclusion Unit 2003).

Making sense of film

An interesting concept here is the influence that movie images have upon our understanding and subsequent perception of mental illness. Norden (1994), focusing upon physical disability in the cinema, illustrates how the movie industry has perpetuated or initiated a number of stereotypes. These stereotypes are regarded as being so durable and pervasive that they have become mainstream society's perception of disabled people and have obscured if not outright supplanted disabled people's perception of themselves. The immense chasm that exists therefore between disabled and screen counterparts is clearly also applicable to a mental health perspective which is reinforced through numerous stereotypes. As Kolker states: '[film] substitutes images and sounds for "real" experience, and with those images and sounds communicates to us and manipulates particular feelings, ideas and perspectives on reality' (Kolker 1988: 14). It can therefore be difficult to determine which aspects viewers are exposed to on the screen actually reflect the real facts regarding mental illness. Further discrimination is provided by viewers who bring their own individual perspective from which they interpret the inputted stimuli. While producers and film-makers might be seen as encoding a single 'meaningful message' to be read by viewers, a sense of polysemic or textual openness applies so that texts are open to more than one possible reading (Moores 1993). There are a variety of factors affecting a viewer's perception here including their prior knowledge and experience that lead to certain viewing perspectives being adopted.

Another core factor concerns the audience member's type of engagement with film and their ability to suspend reality. As Armes states:

> When we watch a film, we make a conscious decision to enter a world of fiction and make believe . . . and place ourselves under the illusory guidance of a maker of narratives. We are not duped or deceived in the sense that we believe we are still in the world of everyday reality, but we do desire to have our emotions aroused and our thoughts provoked.
>
> (Armes 1994: 48)

Allen (1995) refers to this process as *projective illusion* in that viewers know that what they are watching is only an impression of reality yet actively participate in the illusion that cinema affords. This is further argued by Lothe (2000) in the view that fictional film shows us an illusory real world that resembles to the point of confusion the world we know ourselves, a world into which we are free to peep for a couple of hours without participating. The core thread being highlighted here is that of an active spectator voluntarily entering the film world as opposed to a passive viewer having images imposed upon them. It also addresses the notion of a *conscious spectator*, an individual who is able to determine what is real and what isn't. Some of the less obvious fantasy-based material may be harder to determine as manufactured reality. This is especially true when relating to attitudinal qualities or stereotypical content. The problems are caused here when viewers do not have a contrasting point of reality from which to question or challenge what they are exposed to within a particular film. For example, the statistics and facts concerning mentally ill killers do not tie in with the messages being offered by their psychopathic screen counterparts. It is a point made by Gabbard and Gabbard (1999) who indicate that without knowing what the customary behaviour is, the audience has no standard by which to judge the appropriateness of what it witnesses on the screen. In general, the audience member is offered a variety of stereotypical portrayals that fit the popular view concerning mental illness. They are therefore not alerted in many instances to look for different interpretations. An illustration of this can be given with the Necker cube (Figure 7.2), whereby the position of the grey dot changes from the front to the rear of the cube. If not alerted to this fact the viewer can easily miss this dynamic, seeing only one interpretation and not looking further for others.

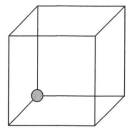

Figure 7.2 The Necker cube.

A further issue here concerns the way in which viewers engage on an emotional level with the medium of film. This is highlighted by Kolker (1988: 14) who states that particular feelings, ideas and perspectives on reality are manipulated through the illusory images that viewers are exposed to. It is certainly the case that what we might challenge on a rational level can be overtaken by what we feel on an emotional one. A classic example of this is the radio broadcast in 1938 by Orson Welles of *War of the Worlds*. The illusory sense of reality created was so powerful that a number of listeners fled their homes for fear of an incoming Martian invasion. The engagement of powerful emotions and subsequent influences upon a recipient's behaviour can also be reflected upon with regard to Brown's (2000) illustration of imitative behaviour in homicides relating to the film *Natural Born Killers* and Russian Roulette deaths relating to the *Deerhunter*. Another consideration is the fact that the sense of trepidation and fear experienced as Freddy Krueger (*Nightmare on Elm Street*) and Michael Myers (*Halloween*) dispatch their victims in grisly fashion can be hard to shake off. It leaves the viewer feeling uneasy and uncertain concerning the real violence potential of the mentally ill, a point not helped by the steady reinforcement through the tabloid media and television drama.

Attraction (connecting with mental health issues)

Of major significance here is the way in which we engage with mental health issues and those portrayed as having mental health problems who generally are not depicted as likable or appealing to the viewer. Our ability to connect with and engage with screen characters is influenced by a number of features that create feelings of attraction. These are illustrated by Hoffner and Cantor (1991) as:

- Liking
- Perceived similarity
- Desire to be like a character

These factors relate to the desirability of the personal characteristics associated with an individual and relate to those that hold positive attributes, are kind and helpful, display positive social and non-verbal behaviours, are successful in coping with threats, and are competent and resourceful. The concept of *liking* is important as it plays a significant part in the type of emotional response evoked in the viewer such as feelings of concern for their welfare. It also engages in the viewer a tendency to feel similar emotions to those experienced on screen (Zillmann 1980). The cinematic world is littered with examples of both likeable and unlikeable mentally ill characters although it is predominantly the latter who seem to be portrayed. Some of those who are liked by viewers can be quite surprising as they even include anti-hero types such as Hannibal Lecter or the murderous Jack Torrance (Jack Nicholson) in *The Shining*. It is heartening, though, to note the greater use of charismatic and attractive stars such as Russell Crowe or Judy Dench who provide the audience with attractive mentally ill role models, a far cry from the stereotypical choices that have proliferated in films of the past. The qualities and characteristics afforded individuals seen on screen are influenced by their perceived attractiveness to the viewer. This is a point addressed by Hatfield and Sprecher (1986) who indicate that physically attractive people are seen as possessing more socially desirable personality traits than unattractive individuals. It is important therefore to present the viewer with a greater number of positive characterisations, thereby helping overall to present a more balanced representation including the portrayal of mentally ill people maintaining relationships, looking *normal* and being engaged with *ordinary* activities.

The sense of engagement with film characters is also strongly influenced by the degree to which we as viewers are able to catch a glimpse of that person's inner world. There are two distinct perspectives that can be taken including:

- *Inside looking out* (internal viewing)
- *Outside looking in* (external viewing)

The first example, *inside looking out*, takes the viewer into the mind of the screen character, offering them a sense of how the world appears from their distinct perspective, whereas the second one, *outside looking in*, locates the viewer firmly at a position external to the character. The ability of film to engage with both of these perspectives is outlined by Rothman who states that: 'Film is a medium limited to surfaces, to the outer, the visible . . . [and yet film is] a medium of mysterious depths, of the inner, the invisible' (Rothman 1988: xv).

There are a number of films presenting directly to us the altered reality of those experiencing mental health problems. An example is the 1960s film *Repulsion* where we are led progressively into a world that is becoming more fragmented and disturbed. It is portrayed very vividly with the hallucinatory imagery of cracks appearing accompanied by strange distorted sounds. As viewers, we are led into experiencing something of Carol's (Catherine DeNeueve) confused world which proves a disconcerting and unnerving experience. Another film, *A Beautiful Mind*, takes the audience member on a journey whereby it becomes unclear as to what is reality and what isn't. It is only later in the film that viewers become aware of the fact that a collection of characters they have been watching are in fact a product of Nash's hallucinatory perspective and are not seen by other people in the film. Ron Howard's direction of this material is cleverly and sensitively handled helping to bring about various feelings in the audience such as confusion, frustration and loss, no doubt similar to those felt by Nash himself. The importance of these types of engagement is the sense of entering into the empathic process of seeing the world from another person's perspective. According to Carl Rogers, accurate empathic understanding means that an individual is completely at home in the universe of another person, sensing that person's inner world of private personal meanings as if it were their own (Kirschenbaum and Henderson 1990). When relating this process to film characters, it is clear that it is a process that will not always be a comfortable one for the viewer and that it will at times prove unsettling and disturbing, especially where a distorted sense of reality is being presented.

The distorted world, however, is not always presented as frightening and destructive as evidenced by the film *Don Juan de Marco*. Here it is depicted as something preferable to the stale and restrictive state that marks reality for a number of people. As viewers we are invited to engage with the fantasy created by Don Juan's (Johnny Depp) world and, along with the psychiatrist Dr Mickler (Marlon Brando), have an opportunity of appraising our own lives and considering the benefits offered by the fantasy existence. This can be considered with regard to Flemming and Manvell's statement that:

> 'Madness . . . provokes fundamental questions about our place in, and understanding of the world. It makes us look more closely at our definitions of the nature of things and at our expectations of what we should follow. Madness, therefore has profound implications for our interpretation of ourselves and of our environment and eventually leads us to question who we are and what we are.'
>
> (Flemming and Manvell 1985: 17)

Film as a medium has much to offer and can provide an extremely impactful engagement with various characters, themes and concepts. Because of this, film has been used for both therapeutic as well as educative purposes. Chaudhuri (2002) illustrates the notion of *Cinematherapy* as a form of self-help in that identifying with characters in films provides the viewer with inspiration as well as opportunities for validation. It relates to the process of vicarious learning through watching someone else encounter similar emotions and experiences. The *film as therapy* theme is further illustrated by Gabbard and Gabbard (1999) who indicate that movies might serve as a 'once-removed' analogue allowing a person to express transference longings that are difficult to verbalise, for example with a phrase such as 'I liked the closeness between therapist and patient in the film'. This makes it therefore an attractive point of reference that can be brought into the therapeutic environment and discussed between client and therapist thereby aiding understanding and insight development. A further application of film is seen in teaching where a comprehension of complex dynamics and issues can be better explored through the use of cinematic examples. This is illustrated by Frisch who asserts that: 'There is no better way to understand nursing clients and their varied psychiatric conditions and diagnoses than by entering into their lives through reading literature or by turning down the lights and experiencing the magic world of film' (Frisch 2001: 782).

There are also a number of educational benefits that can be gained by health care professionals through making film recommendations to students as a means of developing understanding about specific mental health topics (Hyler and Morre 1996; Bhugra 2003). These aspects can be understood in relation to Bandura's (1986) Social Learning Theory in that a complex range of issues can be more easily made sense of by observing them through the behaviour of others. This highlights some of the beneficial qualities offered by the medium of film which, combined with a further development of more realistic and less stigmatising portrayals and a greater involvement with mental health advocates, points the way forward.

Conclusion

As illustrated above, the medium of film impacts upon the viewer through a variety of modes such as imagery, narrative and sound. These, at times, engage their audience in very powerful ways and for a film's duration may deter the actual realisation that what is being viewed is fiction or fantasy. This highlights the potential for engagement with characters, storylines and experiences that in many cases last longer than the ninety minutes or so of a films' screening. The film *Psycho* for example, directed in Hitchcock's inimitable style, has provided a particular way of comprehending and relating to mental illness that enhances our instinctive and primitive fears about difference or the unknown. The association of madness with violence and unpredictability permeates the collective understanding about mental health issues and despite countless heath promotion initiatives over the years, survives as an overall assumption, fuelled by tabloid headlines and colloquial language ('*Psycho*') heard within the media or by one's peers. The cinematic world perhaps in a number of instances is only reflecting the comparative societal view of mental illness as can be seen by looking at historical examples. It does though have the capacity to promote better depictions and views of mental health as demonstrated by films such as *A Beautiful Mind* and *Iris*. This reflects a desire and interest by the public to learn and understand more about the theme of mental illness. As with *A Beautiful Mind*, there may be a touch of voyeurism behind its appeal, although the positive messages being conveyed (attractive role model, the overall sense of survival and conveyance of experience from a felt perspective) all help to construct an overall message that is better suited to educate and develop real understanding about mental illness. While the destructive, psycho-killer type of film will obviously still be produced, the more high-profile positive examples there are to challenge this and reduce the distance felt between the audience member and the topic of mental illness the better.

8   Television

Introduction

One of the core issues concerning the power of television as a communicating medium is the ready accessibility on a daily basis of programmes targeting all interest and age groups. Indeed the range and scope of programmes seem almost limitless, boosted further in recent years with the addition of cable and satellite television providers. There appears to be something for everybody with specific time schedules and programme types geared towards different audiences. There are numerous factors playing a part in how we interact with TV and the subsequent understanding taken away. It may depend to a large extent upon whether we are seeking to be entertained or educated, our levels of interest, as well as the type of programme genre we are watching. Our viewing habits will also play a part with programmes being watched either with full or partial attention. We may be selective, choosing programmes which appeal to us be it one-off shows or serialisations, or alternatively leaving the television on in the background to accompany mundane household chores.

Amidst the myriad of themes or messages portrayed on television are a number of references relating to mental health issues. These references have varying degrees of intention and can be found in even the most surprising genres such as children's TV. There are a substantial number of positive examples to be found although the overall picture reflects that observed in other media sources of having to compete with a mass of stereotypical and stigmatising portrayals. It illustrates the concerns being raised about the predominantly negative portrayal of mental health issues within the media by bodies such as Mind (2000), the Royal College of Psychiatrists (2001) and the Mindout for Mental Health (2001a).

The sender

Influences

When considering the medium of television it is important to examine the influences encountered at the varying stages in a programme's production.

For the purposes of this work, those having an influence over television programmes and the development of messages that are to be transmitted can be regarded as 'shapers'. Invariably the large number of individuals and organisations who have an interest in television programmes presents the potential for conflict because of the differing needs of political, media, health professional and voluntary groups. Each group has its own range of concerns, interests and pressures regarding how particular themes or issues should be depicted. This section focuses upon these 'shapers' and includes the following: political agencies, programme makers, professional groups and service-user groups.

Political agencies

Television programming is subject to a variety of regulatory bodies governing or influencing the way in which they are run. From a European perspective, of particular influence is the European Union (2001) 'Television without Frontiers' directive. Nationally, Ofcom (the regulator for the UK communication industries) has a prime role within the sphere of broadcasting regulation. The Broadcasting Acts of 1990 and 1996 have had a significant impact with the subsequent setting up of the Broadcasting Standards Commission (BSC) and the Independent Television Commission (ITC), both having a regulatory role that concerned matters of taste, decency, fairness and privacy. The BSC, among other things, provided codes of guidance regarding what is covered on television. There is particular reference made to people with disabilities or mental health problems with the statement:

> People with mental health difficulties are [liable to be stereotyped], while words like 'loony', 'nutter' and 'schizo' may cause great offence. Care should be taken not to propagate myths nor to stigmatise. Programme makers should also take care not to add a stereotype, for example to suggest that black people with a schizophrenic illness are invariably black or dangerous. Programmes should seek to avoid stereotypes by consulting with people with mental health difficulties through the production process whenever appropriate.
>
> (BSC 1998: 19)

It is interesting to note that despite these guidelines a large number of programmes subsequently were still found to be carrying negative portrayals of mental health issues. These are invariably defended by programme makers with comments relating to issues such as creative freedom, dramatic appeal or audience expectations. The section within the ITC guidelines concerned with mental health issues stated:

> There is a danger of offence in the use of humour based on physical, mental or sensory disability, even where no malice is present. Reference

to disability should be included only where necessary to the content and patronising expressions replaced by neutral terms.

(ITC 2002: 12)

This is not always clear cut, especially when what is regarded as offensive is defended by programme makers. Notable examples of this include *Brass Eye*'s coverage of a paedophilia storyline and the 'offensive' and insensitive references made to the mentally ill on the *11 O'clock Show*. The programme makers supported their portrayal by pointing out that the show was intended to be satirical and provocative (Brindle 2000).

Both the BSC and the ITC have now had their responsibilities taken up by Ofcom, the body charged by parliament to set standards for the content carried by broadcast media. What is interesting is the relative lack of specific focus upon mental health matters featured within Ofcom's Broadcasting Code (2005) as compared with those created by the BSC (1998) and the ITC (2002). Although carrying statements concerning the coverage of substance abuse and suicide, as well as brief references to 'discriminatory treatment' and 'disability' relating to offensive material, there is little particular emphasis upon mental health issues.

A number of guidelines have been made concerning the coverage of suicide. The Department of Health (2002) in their consultation document *National Suicide Prevention Strategy for England*, set out a number of goals to improve the reporting of suicidal behaviour in the media. This reflected upon evidence that the reporting of suicide can increase the rate especially among people already at risk (Schmidtke and Schaller 2000). One of the main recommendations states that:

'By limiting some aspects of the reporting of suicide and by portraying it in ways which may discourage imitation, the media can make an important contribution to suicide prevention' (DOH 2002: 19). Likewise, Ofcom's Broadcasting Code (2005) stresses the need for methods of suicide and self harm to be excluded from programmes except where they are justified by content. These are welcome statements geared towards a more responsible coverage of suicide through the media. While Pirkis and Blood (2001) found the evidence for a causal association between television portrayal of suicide in fictional programmes and subsequent completed or attempted suicide being only of a moderate consistency, Hawton *et al.*'s (1999) findings were more conclusive indicating that a paracetamol overdose storyline in the hospital drama *Casualty* resulted in an increase of self-poisoning incidents in the following two weeks. They concluded that as well as being associated with an increase in self-harming behaviour, media portrayals also have an influence over the choice of method.

The National Union of Journalists (NUJ) (1999) produced a guide for journalists and broadcasters on the reporting of schizophrenia. This provides a concise, educative guide covering some of the factual elements including the assertion that there is little evidence to support the schizophrenia–violence link. It also calls for the need for accurate reporting and the using of correct terminology. The NUJ (1999) code of conduct Clause 3 states that: 'A Journalist shall strive to ensure that the information he/she disseminates is fair and accurate, avoid the expression of comment and conjecture as established fact and falsification by distortion, selection or misrepresentation' (NUJ 1999). The television news format perhaps is less prone to 'tabloid style' reporting although messages may be distorted through associated cues and the attention given to specific details. Factual news reporters are also targeted through particular campaigns such as the Royal College of Psychiatry's *Changing Minds* and the Department of Health's Mindout for Mental Health (2001a) *Mindshift – a Guide to Open-minded Media Coverage of Mental Health*. These are important and much needed initiatives that call upon the media to shift towards a more productive and less stigmatising portrayal of mental health themes.

Programme makers

Writers involved with television programmes have in mind a structure or a message that will be portrayed once the final production has been completed. They are hampered, though, by a number of factors which play a part in shaping the final message. One of these is what Henderson (1996) refers to as 'narrative pace', where restrictive timescales and the need to meet audience expectations means that characters move more swiftly between illness and health than is realistic. This is a criticism which has been levelled at the soaps as this programme format requires rapidly developing and not static storylines. Another difficulty facing television writers is the fact that the visual portrayal of mental well-being may not be regarded as particularly interesting. Crisis situations can be depicted very powerfully creating maximum impact within storylines. The soaps contain many examples here of mental ill-health adding a touch of spice to storylines such as Jimmy Corkhill's erratic and violent behaviour (*Brookside*/manic depression), Zoe Tate's setting fire to a church and attempted murder (*Emmerdale*/schizophrenia) and Joe Wicks barricading himself in his room as a result of paranoid thoughts (*Eastenders*/schizophrenia). The expectation that this is what the audience want to see is reinforced by McQuail's (1997) view that media organisations and those who work in them develop stereotypes concerning the interests, expectations and cultural tastes of their regular or intended audience and seek to match these stereotypes with appropriate content.

Another core issue regards the extent to which writers engage in research (this term is used very loosely here) in order to find out about the themes being addressed. Arguments in support of researching topics indicate that it affords valuable insights into the material being presented whereas those against maintain it contaminates the act of writing. A more honest excuse perhaps concerning the absence of research is given by a *Brookside* writer who points to the tedious, boring process of attending to factual and technical details (Henderson 1996). This obviously has an influence over the degree of sensitivity and understanding shown towards the subject area being covered. A recent series of Channel 4 drama programmes including *Black Dog* and *Insight in Mind* have been written by individuals who have experienced mental health problems. This brings about an important and refreshing change as topics are handled by individuals who arguably have the greatest levels of insight and understanding.

As regards TV production, what we finally see on TV is the culmination of a complex negotiation process and a multitude of competing pressures. Perhaps the most significant factor influencing the degree of responsibility shown to subjects covered is that of ratings. This is borne out by a *Brookside* producer who says that there is no point in producing challenging storylines unless audiences watch them (Henderson 1996). A major concern facing those involved in producing television programmes is that audiences may switch off, a factor that will no doubt greatly govern the way in which issues are portrayed. Commercial pressures therefore may lead to an increase in dramatic portrayal and a reduction in realism connected to mental health storylines. Another problem within programme making relates to potential bias of the particular perspective of those involved. The type of message sent out is largely dependent upon the predominant view of mental illness among those involved in programme production. This is an important point to note as even the documentary format can be regarded to a certain extent as being constructed and contrived by those making them (Collins 1990). What we are exposed to, therefore, can be seen as having been filtered through the programme makers' view of the world with varying degrees of sensitivity consequently being shown.

Professional groups

When making programmes which involve mental health themes it is interesting to look at the degree of involvement of mental health professionals. Those participating may be chosen either to help with research or to provide 'expert' opinion. As with other subject areas there are a number of familiar faces who have regular involvement with the medium of television. Bourdieu (1996) reflects upon this and the fact that a number of those who speak regularly on television will be virtually on call. Indeed it may be that having known and trusted faces who can be contacted spares researchers a great deal of trouble in locating an appropriate source. Organisations such as the Royal College of Psychiatrists even list topics under which their media experts are listed.

Alongside the BSC (1998) guidelines for contributors (see Figure 8.1), a number of professional bodies such as the Royal College of Psychiatrists and the British Psychological Association (2002) have developed guidelines for their members who appear in the media. Those most sought after to provide comment are seen as the special thinkers, who can think and communicate

Contributors should:

- Be told what the programme is about

- Be given a clear explanation of why they were contacted by the programme

- Be told what kind of contribution they are expected to make – i.e. interview or part of a discussion

- Be informed about the areas of questioning and, wherever possible, the nature of other likely contributions

- Be told whether their contribution is to be live or recorded; and if recorded whether it is likely to be edited

- Not be coached or pushed or improperly induced into saying anything which they know not to be true or do not believe to be true

- Whenever appropriate be made aware of any significant changes to the programme as it develops which might reasonably affect their original consent to participate, and cause material unfairness

- If offered an opportunity to preview the programme, be given clear information about whether they will be able to effect any change in the programme

Figure 8.1 Broadcasting Standards Commission (1998) *Codes of Guidance.*

effectively in these conditions where no one else can do so (Bourdieu 1996). Unfortunately this has meant in most instances selecting health care professionals over service-user groups perhaps demonstrating prejudicial and stereotypical attitudes. This obviously raises a number of issues as those who have experienced mental health problems may be stigmatised against regarding the trustworthiness afforded their accounts.

From a professional perspective, there are a number of well-known faces and voices who have appeared regularly on television and radio speaking about or presenting programmes which have a mental health content. Take for instance Raj Persaud, consultant psychiatrist and programme presenter / 'resident expert' whose popularity within the media has even included appearances on shows such as Channel 4's *Countdown*. In the past, notable 'celebrities' have included Clare Rayner, nurse and agony aunt, as well as the psychiatrist Anthony Clare, who had his own television and radio series *In the Psychiatrist's Chair*. We can see therefore the reassuring nature of turning to these respected and trusted figures for guidance on anxiety provoking stories concerning the mentally ill. In a sense it is a bit like going to the family GP for advice on health matters as they represent an authority we trust in and feel secure with.

The professionals are found in abundant supply on daytime TV (e.g.

Dr Hilary) providing timely advice to callers, viewers and even those present in the studio. Other programmes such as the 'talk shows' usually have a resident expert on hand whose purpose ranges from the provision of sensitive and reassuring comments through to that of promoting their new book which *'fortunately'* they have with them in the studio. Professional 'experts' are even included in reality TV shows such as *Big Brother* where a psychologist's view is offered to help viewers understand the interpersonal dynamics they have been witnessing. An alternative view is that this seems more about trying to convince their audience that these types of show are more than an exploitation of participants for their viewers' entertainment but really can be regarded as valid forms of social experimentation.

Service-user groups

There has been a wealth of criticism directed towards the media concerning the under involvement of a service-user perspective compared to the involvement of professional groups. There is still a stark difference, perhaps because the 'professional voice' is seen to carry greater weight and earns greater respect and trust. However, the need for greater realism in the portrayal of mental health issues has seen service-users (both individuals and groups) having an increased involvement within the media, be it providing 'expert' comment or more directly through programme making as with the aforementioned Channel 4 programmes *Black Dog* and *Insight in Mind*.

An area in which the service-user groups and voluntary organisations are particularly active is in producing guidelines or reports for the media. A significant example of this is the media booklet provided by the Samaritans (1997) relating to the reporting of suicide. Mind in particular has been particularly active in campaigning and research and has compiled the important *Counting the Cost* report (Mind 2000) which highlights stereotypical coverage of mental health issues in the media. Rethink (formerly the National Schizophrenia Fellowship) stresses that the best way to improve media portrayal is to broadcast or print people's direct experience of it (Rethink 2002). A number of its media volunteers have appeared on TV in programmes such as *Newsnight* and *Sky News*. The Zito Trust is also involved in a number of initiatives attempting to enlighten the media regarding the need to respect patients and provide the best kind of therapeutic care possible. The organisation Mental Health Media offers media skills training and information material for users of mental health services and mental health workers (Mental Health Media 2002).

It is interesting to note the link which television stations have with service-user groups. For example, Alison Walsh the Disability Adviser at Channel 4 liaises with programme makers and encourages producers to hire researchers who are disabled or have experience of the issues being covered in the programme. Walsh (2002) stresses that production companies might also show rough cut versions of programmes to service-user groups in order to gauge their reaction and obtain feedback. The initiatives outlined above are very welcome and clearly play a vital part in tempering the more dramatic and unrealistic portrayals which are regarded as more audience pleasing.

The message

As previously addressed, there are a wide range of factors which influence the messages which are to be transmitted. The packaging and shaping of the message to be sent out is largely governed by the particular programme format and its intended audience. It may help to understand this by categorising television programmes into their various types. From a broad perspective we can see programmes either having a fictional or factual base. To some degree this may determine the aim of the message sent out, whether it be to educate or to entertain. Programmes will therefore fall somewhere along the education–entertainment spectrum, either separately or in some instances addressing both poles.

The following section explores a range of fictional and factual programme genres looking at the contrasting ways in which mental health images are portrayed. It focuses in particular upon issues such as characterisation, words and language used as well as the core focus upon either positive or negative imagery.

Factual

News

TV news offers us immediacy and can have a powerful impact upon attitudes with the pictures it brings into our lives. This is starkly illustrated by the stirring and harrowing pictures of starving children, abused and desperate war refugees, bemused and lost survivors of a natural disaster, or the unforgettable horror of the pictures relating to the terrorist attacks on 11 September 2001. These images are so forceful that we are left haunted by them and either feel helpless or compelled to act in some way. We are moved both by the visual cues as well as the emotive words and tone used. This perhaps marks the main distinction between television news and the printed format as stories are brought with greater impact into our living space. As demonstrated within perceptual theory, issues that are brought more forcibly to the forefront of our attention are subsequently harder to relegate to the background (Köhler 1929).

The overly negative and stereotypical coverage of mental health issues is influenced by the placing of emphasis or type of associations made. The predominant message which emerges seems to be that of the mentally ill being an unpredictable and violent group. An example of this can be found in the coverage of high profile murder cases where the perpetrator is later found to be suffering from some form of mental illness. As demonstrated by

Pavlov's (1958) process of classical conditioning, an association between the themes of violence and psychological disorder is made and reinforced on a continued basis thereby evoking a new learned response – that the mentally ill are dangerous. We see the individual with mental health problems primarily in the role of *perpetrator* and not the more appropriate one of *victim*, a fact supported by Mind's (2000) *Counting the Cost* report and the Department of Health's (1999) *Safer Services: National Inquiry into Suicide and Homicide by People with Mental Illness*. It is perhaps the case, therefore, that the difficulties and problems experienced by the mentally ill are not so easily depicted or regarded as being particularly newsworthy. This helps to reinforce the barrier and sense of distance felt from those with mental health problems and it seems that despite the move towards care in the community, many present-day attitudes remain firmly rooted in the past with our fears fuelling a desire to remove 'madness' from society. It is vital that news broadcasters have an appreciation of the total effect generated by their coverage and work towards a more balanced style of reporting promoting the topic *mental health* in equal proportion to that of their own show. News programmes will feel the same commercial pressures as those experienced by the newsprint media, being drawn towards 'audience grabbing' styles of presentation, and the danger is of television genres starting to merge together. This is where the need to entertain and gratify the audience overtakes considerations for educating them, as illustrated recently by the way in which the verdicts in the Michael Jackson trial were shown on Sky News. To all extents and purposes the viewer could have been waiting expectantly to see who would be voted off in the latest reality game show, all sensitivities towards the seriousness of the topic concerned momentarily suspended for a dramatic and suspenseful piece of TV.

Documentary

Documentaries were among those programme types found to be dealing most extensively and sympathetically with mental illness (Wober 1991). They are largely educative in nature geared towards bringing about a greater understanding and acceptance of themes covered. Documentary making is a far from easy process which is highlighted by Bourdieu's (1996) statement that there is nothing more difficult to convey than reality in all its ordinariness. This raises the concern that what we see is not necessarily a genuine representation as programme makers and editors have a vested interest in making documentaries more interesting and appealing to their targeted audience.

There have been a large number of documentaries on television (both single programmes and series) covering mental health issues. Notable series include the BBC's *States of Mind* and *A Living Hell*, Channel 4's *Inside My Head* and *Young Minds*, as well as Channel 5's *Driving Mum Crazy*. What the documentary format importantly allows us is a view of how individuals and their family experience mental health difficulties. It is a connecting experience in that the audience are helped towards a more empathic understanding of the issues being portrayed. For example, *Inside My Head: Michael* depicted a 16-year-old with schizophrenia. The surprise potentially for viewers was in seeing an eloquent, brave and expressive teenager who, despite his worsening condition, continued to express what he was experiencing and feeling. What was shown here reflected a very real glimpse of the suffering not only endured by Michael but also by his family. From an attentional perspective we can see a range of factors being employed within the documentary genre such as the engagement of curiosity and interest as a recipient's desire for greater under-standing is stimulated (Child 2004). The style of presentation is important as it has the capacity to either draw us into the role of detached voyeur or that of engaged and compassionate viewer. The former might be evoked through the choice of mental health issues such as body dysmorphic disorder or Tourette's syndrome that entice the viewer to gawk at those featured in a manner reminiscent of the carnival freak show. The latter style, however, provides opportunities to hear the *sufferer*'s story and for viewers to gain a greater awareness and understanding not only of the condition being highlighted but something of the lived experience as well.

Docu-soaps / reality TV

Over the past few years there has been a rise in the number of programmes shown which fit the docu-soap / reality TV label. This incorporates all the 'fly on the wall' experimental type programmes that provide us with regular glimpses of people going about their daily lives. Whether these 'daily lives' are naturally occurring or in part constructed for them varies. The focus for these shows might be profession based (*Driving School* and *Vets in Practice*), situ-ation based (*Life Laundry, What Not to Wear*), experiment based (*Prisoner: the Experiment*) or game show based (*Big Brother* and *I'm a Celebrity Get Me out of Here*). The impression given from these shows is that the partici-pants do not seem to really matter, and they are coaxed into performing solely for our amusement and entertainment. It is as Woods states, a form of mass voyeurism: 'reality television, a strange land where dignity no longer lives or matters' (Woods 2002).

There are many parallels which can be drawn here with the historical pur-suit of visiting the old asylums in order to observe the 'antics' of the insane. It includes observing the conflicts and emotions that real people endure and either connecting with them through an empathic sharing of effect or remain-ing distanced but entertained by their potentially humiliating experiences. The general impression given by many of these shows is that participants are seen less as feeling people but more as objects to be manipulated and controlled for our entertainment. It conjures up images of *The Truman Show*, a film where the main character's whole life was being directed and manipulated, unbeknown to him, by the television company. These types of show are generally justified on two counts involving entertainment and social experimentation. The concept of entertainment is perhaps a more honest and satisfying explanation than the social study angle, as looking at how people behave in certain situations appears to have no discernible purpose other than to attract viewers. Indeed, *Prisoner: the Experiment* set out to recreate Zimbardo's 1970s social research study which separated volunteers into the roles of prisoners and warders even though the original study was halted after a few days because of the psychological distress encountered by those taking part. Even the entertainment angle does not sufficiently address the issues of active manipulation and public humiliation that are part of this process. Some shows even have a gladiatorial feel with the audience and panel of 'experts' having the power to decide contestants' fates. Examples here include *Pop Idol* and *The X Factor* which show us the visible degradation, ridicule and distress endured by the participants who are voted off, in some cases with extremely unnecessary and hurtful personal remarks being made. We have other shows such as the *Life Laundry* where, fortunately perhaps for the programme makers, participants cry mostly on cue when challenged with the need to throw away objects they have held onto that relate to a deceased relative. Although in part having a connecting quality relating to the audience's opportunity to identify with participants, shows such as these tend to breed a sense of indifference towards the distress of others. The discomfort and suffering of others is presented in a sanitised and detached way with the commercial needs of programme makers and the entertainment needs of the audience taking priority over those of the participants.

Another type of programme worth considering is that concerned with improvement of appearance, lifestyle and environment. The problem with the proliferation of these types of programme is the implied message that we the viewers are satisfying ourselves with imperfection and consequently need to change. As discussed in Chapter 5, the need to strive towards perfection that is reinforced by large sections of the media has a negative and detrimental effect upon many people's self-esteem and body image satisfaction. For example, the resonance caused by Trinny and Susannah's (*What Not to Wear*) critical and caustic scolding of their participant's choice of clothing is perhaps hard to detach from for a number of viewers who subsequently have these remarks reverberating within their own thoughts when selecting items to wear. The very real damage from shows such as these is reflected in a number of studies that demonstrate the impact of television exposure upon body image distortions and the development of an internalised ideal body concept (Myers and Biocca 1992; Martin and Kennedy 1993; Borzekowski *et al.* 2000).

Talk shows

There is currently a proliferation of talk shows on TV, the quality of which varies greatly and certainly covers the full education–entertainment spectrum.

First, we have the more focused and informative subject-based shows such as *Esther* that display a degree of sensitivity towards those taking part who are sharing emotive and vulnerable issues. We also have the studio debate format covering topical issues as seen with shows such as the now defunct *Kilroy*. Perhaps the most popular version, though, is the problem–relationship type show such as *Ricki Lake, Oprah* and *Jerry Springer*. A core feature of all of these shows is the charismatic presenter after whom it is named, clearly informing us the viewer who the most important person is. They demonstrate greatly varied facilitation styles that range from the sensitive and understanding through to the exploitative and abusive.

The exploitation of participants may be regarded almost with a sense of *schadenfreude* where viewers can delight in the mess that those taking part seem to make of their relationships and personal lives. It might be that participants' partners reveal illicit affairs, pregnant lovers or the fact that they are actually trans-sexual. Indeed, shows such as *Ricki Lake* even disclose the results of paternity tests live on air. Apart from a few isolated examples, people's personal and relationship difficulties are served up to the audience in a predominantly unconcerned and insensitive manner. As with the docu-soap/reality TV format the overall impression given is that the needs of those taking part is less important than the entertainment needs of the audience. It is uncertain exactly what the attraction is for those taking part although a study by Rene Diekstra, professor of clinical psychology at Leiden University, suggested that appearing on TV could be regarded as therapy itself (Sheldon 1996). This research has resulted in the Foundation for Mental Health giving advice to programme makers about providing those taking part with written details about the nature of their participation (Sheldon 1996). The extent to which this is carried out or followed up to ensure that details are understood is debatable. Our doubts are perhaps strengthened by the awareness of how important ratings are to the show and the incentives for programme makers to perhaps coerce participants towards levels of disclosure that they are unprepared for. Even within a therapeutic context, disclosing intimate details will feel unsettling and can leave individuals feeling exposed and vulnerable. What then of being led towards this point not at one's own pace but within the time constraints of a television show's schedule, in front of countless numbers of viewers and with the rather false sounding assurance of 'don't worry you'll be offered counselling after the show' ringing in one's ears? It is a shame, therefore, that the therapeutic and educational potential of this format is overshadowed by its entertainment value. If handled sensitively the potential is for these shows to act as on-air self-help groups with those taking part feeling supported and those watching being made more aware of certain issues such as bullying, eating disorders or coping with disability and learning, albeit vicariously by observing those taking part. This promotes the concept referred to by Yalom (1995) as *Universality*, where viewers feel that they are not alone with particular problems and are empowered to seek help. This is complemented by the offering of advice about available resources such as the helpline shown at the end of programmes.

Fictional

Drama

There is an abundance of TV drama shows (particularly police or hospital based) covering mental health issues and providing a mixture of positive and negative portrayals. The depiction though as with many other genres seems to be overwhelmingly negative with many stereotypical characterisations being made. This is highlighted in particular by a study carried out by Wilson *et al.* (1999) exploring the depiction of the mentally ill in prime-time drama (see Figure 8.2). Concerns were raised by the authors that unpleasant, aggressive and antisocial actions are sourced in the characters' mental illness. Persons with a mental illness were constructed as abnormal and unattractively different from the viewer, for example as failures/unproductive, asocial and outcast. This concurs with the findings of Signorielli (1989) who found that characters in prime-time drama portrayed as mentally ill were more likely to be depicted as violent or as victims than any other character. They were also more likely to be portrayed as bad and least likely to be portrayed as good, most being depicted as failures. It is a process that is strongly reflected within labelling theory where the 'deviant' is characterised alongside a set of stereotypical assumptions (Moore 1988).

A drama show that was actually set in a mental health hospital in Glasgow (*Psychos*) attracted a fair degree of criticism concerning its title and portrayal of mental illness. The opening episode highlighted a range of negative associations including the mental illness–violence link, a general detachment between staff and patients, as well as the dubiously unclear psychological state of professional staff involved. One scene which depicts a patient vehemently

---

- Dangerousness-aggressive
- Simple/childlike
- Unpredictability
- Failures/unproductive
- Asocial
- Vulnerability
- Dangerousness-incompetence
- Untrustworthy
- Caring/empathic
- Social outcast

Features listed in order of priority with highest frequency examples placed above

---

Figure 8.2 The depiction of the 'mentally ill' in prime-time drama (Wilson *et al.* 1999).

stressing his rationality but being dismissed by staff members is reminiscent of Rosenhan's (1973) study; 'On Being Sane in Insane Places'. Disappointingly perhaps the patient later returns to stereotype announcing in a ward round, 'I am the rightful King of England'. Popular drama series such as *Casualty* frequently include storylines that involve mental health themes and this hospital drama currently features a mental health nurse as one of the staff team. The dramatic potential of mentally ill characters is perhaps too good to avoid and storylines are often stereotypical and misleading. For example, one episode in particular centred on a mental health group home and highlighted the plight of their tormented neighbour who was unable to sell his home. This in itself would be bad enough but the story continued with some of the group home's residents managing to blow up their house while another committed suicide by laying down on a set of train tracks. Such coverage is obviously geared towards viewers' entertainment and attracting higher ratings. This does not support the statement made in the BBC's (2005) production guidelines that: 'We aim to reflect fully and fairly all of the United Kingdom's people and cultures in our services. Content may reflect the prejudice and disadvantage which exist in our society but we should not perpetuate it' (BBC 2005).

A more balanced and informed coverage of mental health issues is clearly needed as demonstrated through programmes such as Channel 4's drama *Losing it*. This programme located mental health issues within everyday 'normal' experiences presenting characters whom the audience could relate to and identify with. It clearly demonstrated that viewers can be engaged and entertained without having to resort to misleading and incorrect stereotypes.

Soaps

As with the television drama there are many examples where mental health issues have been included within the soaps and it seems as if each show has carried one or more storylines, for example: Shelley Unwin's depression and agoraphobia in *Coronation Street*; Zoe Tate's schizophrenic breakdown in *Emmerdale*; Jimmy Corkhill's manic-depressive episodes in *Brookside*; and Joe Wick's paranoid, psychotic behaviour in *Eastenders*. There is generally a tried and tested soap format although with some differences in the approach. This is observed by Henderson (1996) in relation to the more popular soaps with *Coronation Street* and *Eastenders* being character-driven (not issue-led) whereas *Brookside* is driven by social issues with the aim of provoking debate. Naturally these aspects will play a part in how mental health issues are characterised in the programmes while also being influenced by commercial factors and the intense pressure of developing storylines to maintain existing audiences and attract new ones.

The soaps in particular present us with an array of attractive role models, easily identifiable by the target audience which may have positive as well as negative associations. An example of this can be related to the self-harming storyline in *Hollyoaks* as experienced by the glamorous character Lisa. It is unclear, though, exactly what assumptions or associations might be made here with both positive (glamorous and attractive characterisation) and negative (self-harming behaviour) connections being made leaving viewers to form their own interpretation based upon personal knowledge and experience. This process is highlighted by Livingstone:

> Soap operas cannot offer clear and singular solutions to the personal and moral problems portrayed . . . the complexity and multiplicity of the text invites the viewer to impose a certain order or closure according to his or her own notions of what is likely or desirable or meaningful.
>
> (Livingstone 1998: 52)

The narrative and structure of soaps offer a contrast to traditional shows, which offer a beginning, middle and end, by serving up an endless middle, with narratives weaving in and out of each other, remaining unfinished and full of potential for future development (Livingstone 1998). This is complemented by the presence of between four and seven sub-plots per episode, all relatively independent of each other (Gripsrud 2002). This has a profound influence upon the degree of realism being presented especially in terms of the rapid shift observed between states of wellness and ill health. This is frequently seen with those who are ill either disappearing or making dramatically swift recoveries. What is not often depicted, apart from rare instances such as the wheelchair-user Chris Tate in *Emmerdale*, is a character's prolonged living with disability or illness. This is especially true in the case of mental health problems where characters fluctuate between states of wellness and illness but are not generally shown as learning to adapt and cope with their difficulties. The unrealistic and sensational portrayal of mental illness can in part be put down to the constraints of time and character type, as well as the need to keep viewers engaged by ending on a dramatic note (Livingstone 1998).

Comedy

A study by Wober (1991) found that mental illness was seldom portrayed through comedy shows although, when it did, the depiction was rarely sympathetic. Certain programmes such as *Brass Eye* and the *11 O'clock Show* have been heavily publicised and criticised for what were seen as offensive or insensitive references. It seems that there is scant evidence of positive characterisation in comedy although, on a rare note, the TV sit-com *Takin' Over the Asylum* was praised by mental health service-users as a reasonably accurate and balanced portrayal, depicting psychiatric patients as articulate and humorous (Henderson 1996). This differs from the usual fare which is commonly served up such as the 'escaped from the asylum' situational comedy characterisation. This is the tired old stereotypical format which is used to raise a few laughs as illustrated by Victor Meldrew's plight at being shaved for a hernia operation by an escaped 'mental patient' in the comedy sit-com *One Foot in the Grave*. It seems that another tried and tested formula in comedy shows features characters fearing for their own state of mind. A notable illustration of this can be seen in an episode of *Fawlty Towers – The Psychiatrist* which shows Basil Fawlty's increasingly eccentric and frustrated behaviour when attempting to convince a psychiatrist of his healthy mental health state. This is another example where what is essentially a serious and distressing theme is treated in a casual and dismissive way. Basil Fawlty's desperate need to assert his wellness seems merely to reflect something of the societal need in distancing oneself as far as possible from the scary and unsettling topic of mental illness.

Other depictions seem to highlight notions of craziness or insanity with characters exhibiting zany, eccentric and unpredictable behaviour. These portrayals are mainly stereotypical with depicted behaviour being all too predictable and fitting the expected type. There are many examples of this in classic comedy shows such as Spike Milligan's *Q* series or *Monty Python's Flying Circus*, which famously featured a sketch about 'loony party' election candidates. As discussed in Chapter 7, a major issue with regard to whether or not a comedic representation is offensive or not concerns the way in which audience members are engaged, either laughing *at* or *with* those being depicted. An interesting example here concerns an ongoing sketch running through consecutive episodes of the comedy show *Little Britain*. This featured Anne, a care in the community patient whose clearly inappropriate behaviour (e.g. urinating in ponds and throwing unwrapped loaves of bread at ducks) allied with the total lack of awareness by her accompanying psychiatrist seemed to poke as much fun at those with mental health problems as it did to the system set up to care for them. The culmination of these sketches seemed to illustrate that Anne's eccentric and bizarre behaviour was assumed, perhaps reflecting Thomas Scheff's (1968) assertion of the mentally ill behaving according to expectation. What is clear is that viewers will have their own individual thoughts about what they are watching. The perspective from which material is viewed will help determine how characters are engaged with, and, for example, whether or not we are amused by the strange antics of the mentally ill or alerted to the overly stigmatising societal response or the deficits in care.

Children's TV

A study by Wilson *et al.* (2000) found 46 per cent of children's television programmes surveyed containing references to mental illness. These references particularly related to vocabulary and characterisation with words including terms such as 'crazy', 'mad', 'losing your mind', 'wacko', 'cuckoo' and 'loony'. They noted in particular the opening song to Tiny Toon adventures which begins: 'We're tiny, we're toony, we're all a little loony . . .' The characterisation was interesting with individuals being placed into two sets: the comic character, displaying illogical and irrational actions; and the evil villain, determined and obsessive. Their physical attributes and behaviours were commonly exaggerated, denoting and marking these characters as being different. What is surprising is the extent of programming within this particular genre that carries content relating to mental health issues. This reaffirms the findings of Scheff (1968) who sees our stereotyped imagery of mental health issues being learned in early childhood and continually reaffirmed inadvertently in ordinary social interaction. It is the predominance of negative and misrepresentative characterisation that is particularly disturbing and which clearly signals the need for a greater number of positive and more realistic imagery. Children therefore are frequently exposed to the message that mental illness either represents a threat or is an object of ridicule. This helps to create a negative mindset which serves to obstruct the receipt or perception of messages dealing with mental illness in a more accurate and sympathetic way. As identified in educational workshops run as part of the Mental Health Awareness in Action programme, a significant degree of learning about mental health issues comes from the media (Pinfold 2003). Potentially, what is needed is an increase in programmes that feature more productive examples and present role models with whom viewers are able to identify, such as the storylines in *Grange Hill* covering issues of teenage pregnancy and bullying. It is this type of portrayal that is important, holding difficult issues up for closer inspection and tackling aspects that may otherwise remain largely unexpressed.

The recipient

Making sense of television

A number of theoretical approaches such as personal construct theory, Gestalt theory and schema theory address our predisposition to learn and interpret messages in specific ways. From a personal construct theory perspective we each have a unique way of seeing the world around us which is governed by our own personal constructs. These constructs are borne out of past experience and are constantly being tested out, refined and revised in light of subsequent experience (Epting 1984). Gestalt theory looks at how incoming sensory stimuli are processed and organised into what is regarded as a meaningful and unified whole (King and Wertheimer 2005). Alternatively our base of understanding and interpretation may be related to our cognitive schemas. Schemas can be understood as patterns which are imposed on a complex reality or experience in order to assist in explaining it (Piaget 1958). These schemas are constructed in relation to a stock of shared social experiences (Shore 1996) and include attitudes and emotions (Höijer 1998).

What the above theoretical approaches have in common is the influence that past experience has in predisposing us to interpret stimuli from a certain perspective and how this affects the way we subsequently make sense of things. For example, the Gestalt process of closure relates to the way in which we take what is initially incomplete and fill in the gaps, rounding off messages to create our own understanding (Hamlyn 1957). There are a number of issues which predispose us to see things from a particular perspective. A study by Gunter and Wober (1992) illustrates how our cultural base may influence our perception and cites examples of how American and British audiences differed in terms of viewing scenes on television either negatively or positively. From these arguments the inference seems to be that the actual framing of the transmitted message is a secondary issue to the individual's own base for understanding things from a certain perspective. This is supported by Livingstone who states that: 'The active viewer makes sense of programmes relatively unconstrained by the structure of the text, drawing instead upon his or her interests, knowledge and experience' (Livingstone 1998: 37).

Philo (1990) contests the view that what we see and understand is conditioned by pre-existing assumptions. He argues that our beliefs may have contradictory elements in them and that our perception is not insulated against the processes by which people try to win our consent to see the world in a given way. In Philo's (1990) study, the extent to which subjects believed in the television version of the world depended on several factors, particularly on whether they had access to alternative accounts. This is an important point which is reflected in Höijer's (1998) research where meaning is seen as being created by a network of relations between the text, audience, social reality and other texts seen or due to be seen. The sense we make of television is very much an individual experience, largely influenced by the unique way in which we, as individuals, think and the ways in which we perceive the world around us. Murdock (1998) highlights the significant difference between fiction and news genres when it comes to how well texts are understood. In particular she found that the reception of news events is often quite brief and sketchy, sometimes fragmentary and not as coherent and elaborate as the reception of fiction. What is particularly unsettling about this is the assertion that television news is our main source of information for national and international events (Philo 1990). Murdock (1998) postulates that it may be the case that fiction is easier to interpret because it is closer to the narrative mode – a story-based mode that deals with a sequence of events, characters and happenings. These have dramatic qualities (and some moral point) whereas news follows the more difficult paradigmatic mode, based on a more scientific way of thinking in which logical reasoning and concept formation play important roles.

Naturally television presents us with a rich medium for receiving messages and subsequently testing out and revising assumptions, thoughts or ideas. The proliferation of negative characterisation and stigmatising imagery presents a depressing picture regarding potential change. Audience reception research, though, has shown people's ability to challenge incoming messages.

As Kitzinger (1999) states, people can consume different messages and may also challenge one representation by drawing on another. This ability to discriminate and challenge what is being presented relies upon the availability and accessibility of more positive imagery. The ability to discriminate perhaps lies at variance with the statement in the Newson report (Barker 2001) that 'The principle that what is experienced vicariously will have some effect on some people is an established one and is the reason why millions of pounds are spent on advertising' (Barker 2001).

It is a stance which is contended by Barker and Petley (2001), who point out that the assumption from campaigners, that because TV has some influence it must be the influence they ascribe to it, does not take heed of the myriad of influences which make us laugh or cry, those which interest us or those which prove thought provoking. Television has a responsibility here in what M. Bragg (2001) highlights as a key issue, that of helping people orient towards and understand what it is they are encountering. This should be applied to both negative and positive portrayals of mental health issues and understanding what it is that makes this imagery productive or destructive. An example of this can be related to *The 11 O'clock Show*, a satirical comedy programme which was branded as offensive particularly because of a reference made to 'mentals sitting in their own shit'. The point where perhaps satire misses the mark is summed up by the director of the training and support group Mental Health Media who stated that:

> It is high time that self styled satirists paused for thought. Satire and irony are based on the fact that the majority of people understand you are not being serious, but public understanding of mental health problems is not yet at the level that it is clear that . . . it is satire.
>
> (Brindle 2000)

The message here is that ignorance and lack of awareness provide a ready supply of fuel for discriminating and stigmatising approaches and that what is needed is a greater attention upon education and awareness-raising. This certainly fits in with initiatives such as the Mindout and Changing Minds media awareness campaigns.

Interaction with TV

An important factor influencing our understanding of messages being transmitted is the way in which we interact with television. On the one hand Hobson (1988) asserted that viewers were active rather than passive during viewing, that they were involved and not bored by programmes, and that they were critical rather than mindlessly accepting them. In contrast Barwise and Ehrenberg (1988) describe television as a 'low involvement' medium involving passive activity, mainly watched as a *filler* when we have nothing better or more important to do. They saw the degree of attention required for television viewing as being at a comfortable level. These contrasting viewing styles are outlined by Rubin (1984) who categorised different possible motivations for viewing into broadly active/instrumental (seeking knowledge, reality orientation, social utility) and passive/ritualised (habitual, mindless viewing). Our motivation for active viewing is influenced by our desire for information. This can be seen in particular following a high profile news event such as an abduction and murder case and our desperate need to make sense of what has happened. This need is driven by wanting to understand something of the murderer's mental health state and has the effect of actively 'tuning' us in to what is being presented. We can also reflect upon dramatic storylines covered in the soaps, for example Joe Wick's psychotic breakdown in *East-enders* or Lisa's self-harming behaviour in *Hollyoaks* which grab viewers' attention moving them from passive to active viewing. This is clearly summed up by Nelson:

> The very best in TV drama makes you think. It stops viewers in their tracks, drawing their attention away from the knitting, the newspaper, the distractions of domesticity, to command attention. After the event it plays on people's minds. By coming from an angle different from the regular perspective, by framing things just off-centre, it demands that viewers see something afresh and perhaps to recognise that their accustomed mythologies are inadequate accounts of the world.
>
> (Nelson 1997: 156)

Another issue worthy of consideration is the degree of interaction which viewers have with characters on television. Rosengren and Windahl (1989) distinguished a number of different kinds of 'television relations' including:

- *Interaction* – having the feeling of interacting with actors on the screen
- *Identification* – variable degree of involvement with media figure

Indeed, this can be viewed in terms of parasocial relations where viewers experience interactions between characters as if they themselves were participants, retaining their identity and playing against the characters, taking sides, answering back and reacting emotionally (Horton and Wohl 1956). Livingstone (1998) sees this occurring strongly in drama and soap operas where the relationship is one of connection and of having the feeling of engaging with real people. The importance here is the ability to relate meaningfully with characters, experiencing understanding and sympathy for them. Viewers recognise and identify with the characters and experience them as real people, almost as if they were part of their family (Livingstone 1998). It is this relationship with familiar television characters that Gauntlett and Hill (1999) focus upon when documenting the findings of a five-year British Film Institute project exploring respondents' lives, their television watching and the relationship between the two. In particular, for some respondents, television was seen to bring 'friends' to their living space or indeed even 'one of the family'. It was not seen as just a piece of furniture but meant a lot to respondents, offering information, entertainment and engagement with presenters or actors. Our levels of engagement with characters will be dependent on the type of characterisation being portrayed. Trevor Jordache's abusive and violent character in *Brookside* will no doubt have a significantly different impact on viewers compared to the schizophrenic breakdown of Zoe Tate observed in *Emmerdale*. A major difference here is that Trevor Jordache was depicted from the beginning as a brutal and unlikable character whereas Zoe Tate was somebody whom audiences had first seen and got to know and connect with in a well state.

The way in which we identify with television characters has an affective component as well as a cognitive one. Feshbach and Feshbach (1997) point out that there may be a blurring of the distinction between drama and real experience and that an emotion-arousing event happening to another person will elicit a similar feeling in an observer. On a positive note, this vicarious sharing of affect can help to develop empathy with characters. It has the impact of 'tuning' viewers in to the feelings of those we are watching. From a more critical perspective, we can consider the voyeuristic and exploitative quality of a number of programmes such as the talk shows *Jerry Springer* and *Trisha* having a questionably less than caring approach to those taking part. This can also be applied to documentaries such as the *Driving Mum Crazy* Channel 5 series which was criticised by McClure (2000) as being poorly balanced, suggesting that the purpose of the series was to shock viewers with severe examples of juvenile behaviour. He questions whether this series simply facilitated voyeurism, stating the need to get the balance between informing and entertaining. Likewise, Channel 4's *Witness: 'Valkenberg'* presented a 'fly on the wall' view of the wards in a South African hospital. As McKenzie (1994) states, there was only a superficial coverage of issues and this documentary became more of a voyeuristic process and was always likely to descend into a Victorian freak show.

From this viewpoint, we can see the relationship of television with mental health issues as being a predominantly negative one. Clearly what is needed are stronger and more realistic role models whom we are able to connect with and relate to. For instance the admission by Princess Diana about her struggles with bulimia led to a greater understanding and acceptance of the condition. From a social learning perspective (Bandura 1986), we can see the public was presented with a role model whom they not only could relate to but, in particular, with somebody they had a desire to help and understand. Television drama and soaps in particular present viewers with role models whom they can get to know and identify with. There is a considerable potential here for understanding and awareness raising of mental health issues, although much depends upon the degree of realism and sensitivity being employed. The importance of having access to specific experiences through the medium of television is outlined by Berry and Asamen (1993) who observe that few non-disabled people know individuals with disabilities well enough for information to be shared with them as intimate as that revealed by those on screen. This highlights the educative potential of television as well as the degree of responsibility that programme makers need to demonstrate as there are many examples where the public are actually misinformed through ambiguous and inaccurate depictions.

Television and behavioural change

A great deal of research has been carried out into investigating media effects, focusing upon the impact that television content has upon the subsequent behaviour of viewers. In particular a number of studies have focused upon the link between television content and its subsequent impact upon violent behaviour (Gauntlett 2001). As Livingstone (1998) observes, as well as looking at resultant behaviour, media effects are also concerned with thoughts, emotions, social interactions and attitudes. The media effects model itself has met with considerable criticisms including the implied presumption that the media presents one singular and clear-cut message which viewers are not able to respond differently to or come up with their own interpretations (Gauntlett 1995). Gauntlett further states that the effects model can only really make sense to people who consider popular entertainment to be a set of very basic propaganda messages flashed at the audience in the simplest terms. In Comstock *et al.*'s (1978) model, the act or behaviour seen on television will have an impact on the individual viewer, depending on the degree of positive value attached to the act and on the degree to which it is shown to be close to real life. Therefore, the further removed from reality a television portrayal is, the less likely it is seen to have relevance to the viewer (McQuail and Windahl 1993). Whether or not the viewer perceives portrayals to be unrealistic is debatable as familiar stereotypes or recognisable screen characters may be taken as true to life.

We may regard the link between the media and society as a cyclical one, as each in turn plays a part in shaping the views and behaviour of the other. Television is a particularly influential media source which not only portrays societal trends but can have a direct effect upon individual or societal attitudes. This is highlighted by S. Bragg (2001) who states that television is not so much a window on the world as a mirror and in some ways the maker of society, enforcing attitudes, manners and fashions. This view is also supported by Fiske and Hartley (1978) who indicate that our attitudes are in part shaped by the environment of significance that we have collectively produced. They see part of that environment as comprising the constant stream of 'secretions' that emanate from the small screen. In this sense television can be regarded as being firmly entwined with changes and developments in society.

What perhaps has not been sufficiently addressed is the individual's reaction to media coverage as influenced by personal experiences of mental health problems. Scheff (1968) looks at the extent to which the behaviour of people who are labelled mentally ill is influenced by stereotypical expectations and may be modelled upon characterisations learned through the media. The overwhelmingly negative portrayal of mental health issues in the media plays a part in highlighting the 'deviance' element and reinforcing the effects of labelling. The effects upon the individual and how they perceive themselves can be reflected in the term 'The looking glass self' which illustrates how identity is built primarily as a result of how others act towards and respond to us (Moore 1988). This obviously plays a central part in how individuals experiencing mental health problems subsequently behave. A further consequence is the reaction of others and a failure to adequately connect with the lived experience, treating the individual's actions in light of their underlying psychopathology (Goffman 1963). As illustrated in the Changing Minds campaign (RCP 2001), people with mental health problems have been locked away from society for centuries, but today negative attitudes lock them out more subtly but just as effectively. This all fuels the negative, downward spiral whereby those who are labelled mentally ill embark upon what Becker (1964) describes as a deviant career. Television depictions of mental health issues as a whole play a central role in this process by perpetuating and reinforcing negative, unrealistic and stereotypical imagery.

Modifications in attitudes are governed by the degree of personal motivation we have to change. As Petty and Priester (1994) state, information will only be successful in producing enduring changes in attitude and behaviour if people are motivated and able to process the information, and if this processing results in favourable thoughts and ideas. From a mental health perspective people influenced may lack the necessary skills or self-confidence to translate new attitudes into action. The Dutch critical viewing project explored the influence of television on children's attitudes and beliefs (Vooijs and Van der Voort 1993). The suggestion made was that TV offers a distorted view which can be corrected by comparing it with what happens in real life. This may prove difficult, though, especially where fears or fantasies may be involved. Fears and fantasies can be played upon, for instance as expressed in the comment 'I know that the mentally ill do not pose a significant risk but I still wouldn't allow my children near them'. This is where our primitive instincts prove stronger than our cognitive understanding of reality. Philo's (1990) study found that the fear generated by media accounts was such that it could overwhelm direct experience in formation of beliefs. An example given was the extreme anger shown by the public towards the nanny in *Coronation Street*, Carmel, a character who was sexually obsessed with Martin, the baby's father. The level of emotion aroused seemed to relate to a real event experienced by the viewer and not a fictional account that was observed on screen.

Future needs

What has been highlighted by the above are the many competing and contradictory factors which play a part in what we take away from the messages we are exposed to on television. It seems that despite the multitude of guidelines directed towards television programming there is still an overwhelmingly negative and stereotypical portrayal being used. The vast number of issues covered are presented through a variety of television genres which have a factual or fictional base. The potential for education and awareness-raising is not always realised as entertainment and the pressure of ratings play a significant part. What is clearly needed is a greater input into following up the themes and issues raised. Having brought mental health issues to the public's attention and awareness there is then a great opportunity to 'fill in the gaps' and educate viewers in a meaningful way. Whether the programme has a factual or a dramatic base should not deter it from following up with various messages relating to education or support giving. This has been well applied in soaps, drama programmes and talk shows covering sensitive issues such as sexual abuse, bullying and specific mental health conditions.

There is a need to help viewers discriminate between what are productive and healthy mental health images and what are not. Importantly this is already being done through the increasing recognition which is now being given to the positive and sensitive handling of mental health issues (e.g. the mental health media awards) and the attention drawn towards stigmatising media depictions by Mind's (2000) *Counting the Cost* report or the Royal College of Psychiatrists' (2001) Changing Minds campaign. A welcome addition is also the greater voice and representation being given to mental health user groups/organisations, not only through their direct media involvement but also through their increased influence on mental health legislation. The more that media depictions of mental health issues are shaped by those who best understand them, the greater the opportunity that attitudes and awareness will be changed for the better.

Conclusion

As with print media, it seems that the most popular products offered by the medium of television carry portrayals that on the whole are stigmatising, unrealistic and misleading. This can be seen with genres that have a prime function of entertainment such as soaps, drama and comedy. The job of informing and educating the public about mental health issues remains largely within the news and documentary formats. There have been some welcome attempts over recent years though to marry the educational to the entertaining which bring a number of benefits in the promotion of better understanding and awareness concerning the reality about certain mental health issues. The success of some of these ventures, notably the improved coverage within some of the more popular soaps, has been greeted with praise by mental health advocates and recognised by various mental health awards. Critics might point though towards overly dramatic scenes or depictions that are still present as being on the whole, unrepresentative of the mental health state concerned. At the same time, programme makers might defend this as gearing their material to the needs and desires of their targeted audience, a fact supported by the increase in ratings following a particularly dramatic storyline. This is in a sense sold as the '*pay off*', the price for using their high-profile vehicle (television programme) to carry a particular message. Because the potential benefits are so valuable (high exposure, better education and understanding, a sense of identification with known and liked characters, clear comprehension of the felt and lived experience concerning certain mental health states, feelings of connection with others and further contact information), it is an area where continued development is evidently required. In order to facilitate this, further liaison between programme makers and mental health advocates needs to be fostered. This would help to provide television personnel with clear and definite information, not only of the reality concerning different mental health states but also the impact that poor coverage has upon the lives of those involved. The core message to convey to those involved within television is that coverage need not be totally purged of dramatic content or made so blandly unappealing that mental health issues are no longer showcased. The greater sensitivity now being afforded other historically stigmatised groups (i.e. race / physical disability) is something that needs to be matched by the way in which the mentally ill are treated. Progress has been made although ongoing attention to the promotion of better mental health coverage is clearly required.

9 The Internet

The Internet: the medium

The advent of new media and the Internet offers a rich and valuable resource from which to obtain information. The almost limitless scope of material available and instantaneous access make it an extremely effective source for updating. Evidence-based information, contact details, chat rooms, e-mail, self-help organisations and online therapy are only a few services offered through this new medium. Indeed, it offers a valuable resource not only to health care professionals but also to mental health service-users and other interested parties. From a mental health perspective there is a rich array of resources to choose from. This encompasses a vast selection of Internet sites provided by an extremely diverse selection of organisations and individuals. While this multi-perspective presents those accessing information with a greater selection of choice, it can also make it a bewildering and confusing process. The quality of information varies dramatically from site to site; from credible to unreliable, helpful to harmful and informative to misleading. Although there are various guides and indicators as to which are the more productive sites, the difficulty in distinguishing between the good and poor ones is a matter of some concern. Those accessing the Internet may struggle, therefore, to authenticate the information they find. There are no guarantees regarding the intention or credibility of many individuals or organisations posting information, and in a number of cases this has proved to be harmfully misleading or actively encouraging self-destructive behaviour. Searching the Internet does on the whole present individuals with what could be regarded as a storehouse of treasure although the 'trinkets' clearly have to be sifted out from the piles of accompanying junk. These difficulties are further reinforced by information overload caused by the almost limitless supply of material available.

The Internet does provide a number of benefits and advantages over other information systems. One of the attractions of this new medium is the potential for increased access to health care information for both professionals and health care consumers (Hebda *et al.* 1998; Tomaiuolo 1995; Christensen and Griffiths 2000). It is a fast, accessible and relatively cheap medium that as well as educating offers the potential for empowering mental health service-users. The importance of the Internet as a vehicle for accessing health information is endorsed by the findings that this is one of the most common reasons for using the Internet (Powell and Clarke 2002). It is also an excellent resource for obtaining up-to-date information (Hebda *et al.* 1998), which gives it a clear advantage over that of books. New postings on the Internet replace existing material, whereas new editions of books are brought out while older versions are still available (Scrivener 2002). The currency and speed of updating information online has a great advantage over books which are, in a sense, out of date even before they are published (Booth 2002). Overall, it is a medium that has numerous attractions as well as limitations although these are largely dependent upon the nature of the person accessing material online.

Beginnings

From its conception, there was little indication that the Internet would become as successful and as significant a means of mass communication as it has clearly become. One current estimate reflects that over 10 per cent of the world's population and over half the population of the Western nations now use the Internet (European Information Society Group 2004). In a sense the heralding in of the Internet reflects the experience of cinema in the early nineteenth century and television in the 1950s in the excitement surrounding the huge potential of a new and exciting communicating medium. Its origins date back to the 1960s and the development of packet-switching technology, which entailed breaking strings of data down into small pieces or packets which were then reassembled at their destination (LaBruzza 1997). It was originally used as a US military communications system and was later extended into the world of academia (Graham 1999). Initially, it was limited to just four networked computers joined together but was boosted by the development of a 'hyper-text link' by scientific researchers in Switzerland, allowing an indefinite number of computers to be interconnected electronic- ally. By January 2001, up to 110 million host computers were connected to the Internet with almost 28 million websites accessible (Cooke 2001). A recent study by Ofcom (2004) has estimated that 50 per cent of homes in the UK have Internet access. This trend is set to continue with ongoing developments in technology and enhanced accessibility through means such as mobile phones or television sets.

Regulation and guidance

There is a certain degree of censorship applied to material found on the Internet, for example with content that is deemed to be harmful to children, inciting racial hatred, pornographic or overly violent. Despite some of these initiatives, the Internet remains a largely unregulated medium with numerous perspectives of all quality types finding representation. In some instances an element of self-regulation will be applied, as the organisations or bodies posting material (for example the Royal College of Psychiatrists or the Nursing and Midwifery Council) provide information that is acceptable within the bounds of their specific professional codes of conduct. The majority of sites accessible over the Internet are offered by largely unknown or uncertain sources, a number of which do not come under any external regulation. Some of the problems with regulating the Internet medium are found in the sheer scale and size of this resource. As McQuail (2005) indicates, the Internet is comprised of a network of internationally, interconnected computers and, unlike other media sources, is not owned, controlled or organised by any single body. This means that any attempt at censoring or limiting what can be expressed is met with a sizeable degree of opposition including organisations that advocate freedom of speech. Part of the reason why the Internet has flourished with a minimum of regulation is due to its place of origin: the United States, a country that provides specific constitutional protection for freedom of speech (House of Commons 2001). The globalisation of Internet resources has added further difficulties in censoring or regulating material as what might be banned in one country can be easily distributed from another where such activity is not illegal (Christensen and Griffiths 2003). The mechanics of banning material can be a crude process and the blocking of material that carries sexual content, for instance, can also result in impeding health information concerned with sexually transmitted diseases. As a consequence of the size, easy accessibility and diversity of material available on the Internet, policing this medium is an extremely complex and problematic process. It means that the large discrepancy regarding the reliability and credibility of information posted will be maintained and that alongside many excellent sites will be those that contain misinformation and are potentially dangerous (Morahan-Martin and Anderson 2000).

The British government believes that a distinct regulatory approach to the Internet is required and proposals were made within the Communications Act (2003) to give Ofcom (the regulator for the UK communication industries) the responsibility for 'maintaining content standards in the electronic media'. Ofcom, the Office of Communications is a body set up to regulate the telecommunications services and is becoming progressively involved with the regulation of Internet content. This is much needed, especially with a medium where so many diverse and different types of quality are available. Certainly, various pieces of legislation aid this process, for example the Protection of Children Act (1978), the Sex Offences Act (2003) and the Obscene Publications Act (1964). This picture is complemented by the range of services and resources that guide Internet users as to the 'quality' or 'reliability' of online material. One such method is the provision of kitemarks, logos or seals of quality. An example of this is the Internet Content Rating Association (ICRA), which is an international, non-profit organisation of Internet leaders working to make the Internet safer for children while respecting the rights of content providers. Application of the ICRA label to suitable sites provides them with a 'mark' of acceptable content.

Those searching for health care information have a number of available resources to help guide them towards various products. As with conducting a search through other sources such as academic journals and books, reviewers gain confidence from the type of publication accessed and its academic credibility. To some degree the reliability of sources may be identified through the Journal Citation Reports (an essential, comprehensive and unique resource tool for journal evaluation) or whether the publishers of the books are respected in the field of academic publishing. From a health care perspective, certain titles like the *British Medical Journal* or the *Advanced Journal of Nursing* reassure readers that the articles contained will be quality ones because both are highly respected peer reviewed academic journals. What those searching the Internet require is some means of evaluating the significance or credibility of information being looked at. To some degree this is aided through the association with recognised and credible names, bodies and organisations. For example, if looking for information concerning suicide, one might feel more secure with material found on sites posted by the Samaritans, Department of Health or Royal College of Psychiatry than that located within personal sites or unknown organisations.

Other means exist to select and recognise quality pieces of information such as the availability of evidence-based search tools or the application of kitemarks. While this is to be applauded, the global accessibility of information and the fact that different countries have their own approaches to health care means that there will be potential problems with regard to regulating kitemarks. This is indicated by Thede (1999) who observes that what is appropriate in one country may not be in another. It raises the question as to who would be able to regulate properly the various kitemarks applied, with the WHO (World Health Organisation) being put forward as a potential choice. Some recent developments have moved to provide those searching the Internet with a guide to those sites where information posted has a degree of reliability and can be supported by relevant evidence. Examples of this include the European project WRAPIN (Worldwide Online Reliable Advice to Patient and Individuals). This project provides checks on the reliability of documents posted against established benchmarks and provides evidence if information exists in published literature. The Internet Service Providers Association (ISPA) was established in 1995 and is the UK's trade association for providers of Internet services. As a trade association, membership is voluntary but the companies who choose to become members of ISPA must abide by their UK *Code of Practice* if they are to be able to gain the ISPA UK logo as a mark of commitment to good business practice. The ISPA *Code of Practice* (2002) covers various aspects including legality and decency with regard to content. While there are no specific references to disability discrimination or mental illness, Clause 2.4 (Honesty) could be related to material that is misrepresented or inaccurate:

2.4.1 Members shall use their reasonable endeavours to ensure Services (excluding Third Party Content) and Promotional Material are not of a kind that are likely to mislead by inaccuracy, ambiguity, exaggeration, omission or otherwise.

The MedCIRCLE and MedCERTAIN projects are complementary semantic web projects with the overall objective of developing and promoting technologies able to guide consumers to trustworthy health information on the Internet. The aim is for consumers to be able to 'filter' accessed material more effectively and therefore positively select high quality health information on the web. Further regulation is offered by the Swiss Health on the Net foundation (HON) for the provision of authoritative, trustworthy web-based medical information. The Health on the Net Code of Conduct (Hon Code) was issued in July 1996 to help standardise the reliability of medical and health information available on the worldwide web. This code defines a set of voluntary rules designed to help a website developer practise responsible self-regulation and to make sure a reader always knows the source and the purpose of the information he or she is reading. These guidelines cover the following:

1) *Authority*
Any medical or health advice provided and hosted on this site will only be given by medically trained and qualified professionals unless a clear statement is made that a piece of advice offered is from a non-medically qualified individual or organisation.

2) *Complementarity*
The information provided on this site is designed to support, not replace, the relationship that exists between a patient/site visitor and his/her existing physician.

3) *Confidentiality*
Confidentiality of data relating to individual patients and visitors to a medical/health Web site, including their identity, is respected by this Web site. The Web site owners undertake to honour or exceed the legal requirements of medical/health information privacy that apply in the country and state where the Web site and mirror sites are located.

4) *Attribution*
Where appropriate, information contained on this site will be supported by clear references to source data and, where possible, have specific HTML links to that data. The date when a clinical page was last modified will be clearly displayed (e.g. at the bottom of the page).

5) *Justifiability*
Any claims relating to the benefits/performance of a specific treatment, commercial product or service will be supported by appropriate, balanced evidence in the manner outlined above in principle 4.

6) *Transparency of authorship*
The designers of this Web site will seek to provide information in the clearest possible manner and provide contact addresses for visitors that seek further information or support. The Webmaster will display his/her E-mail address clearly throughout the Web site.

7) *Transparency of sponsorship*
Support for this Web site will be clearly identified, including the identities of commercial and non-commercial organisations that have contributed funding, services or material for the site.

8) *Honesty in advertising & editorial policy*
If advertising is a source of funding it will be clearly stated. A brief description of the advertising policy adopted by the Web site owners will be displayed on the site. Advertising and other promotional material will be presented to viewers in a manner and context that facilitates differentiation between it and the original material created by the institution operating the site.

Some of the aspects identified in the Hon Code are important as they help provide those accessing particular sites with a degree of assurance. Core points raised here relate to transparency of authorship and sponsorship as it may be unclear as to who is actually posting information and what their credentials are. For example, one might feel more reassured in accepting advice about treatment options from a recognised medical practitioner. It is also important to recognise the potential influence from other parties providing sponsorship such as that from pharmaceutical companies. It is particularly alarming, however, to note the number of sites which do not post relevant details. A study by Hersch, Gorman and Sacharek (1998) investigating the quality of health information via the web found that over 80 per cent gave no authorship credentials, 69 per cent were without any indication of author and less than 18 per cent provided the date of posting or upgrading. While checklists, kitemarked sites and evidence-based lists provide those searching for information with a helpful guide, there are some difficulties and limitations involved. Of the many checklists and rating tools available, there are few details about how they have been developed and the criteria used in rating sites. Jadad and Gagliardi (1998) examined 47 instruments used to rate health information websites and concluded that many incompletely developed instruments exist on the Internet and that it is unclear if these tools measure what they intend to measure or whether they cause more harm than good.

With regard to material concerning mental health, there are a number of other useful search bases that include:

Cochrane library (http://www.cochrane.org/index0.htm)
The Cochrane Collaboration is an international non-profit and independent organisation, dedicated to making up-to-date and accurate information

about the effects of health care readily available worldwide. It produces and disseminates systematic reviews of health care interventions and promotes the search for evidence in the form of clinical trials and other studies of interventions. It includes several systematic reviews on mental health topics.

NeLH (National Electronic Library for Health) http://libraries.nelh. nhs.uk/mentalHealth/

This is a mental health specialist library website that only includes information which is deemed reliable, unbiased and relevant. It contains the best available evidence to support people who are making mental health care related decisions. At present this includes NICE guidelines and technology appraisals, Cochrane systematic reviews, and a range of best practice articles (including clinical evidence chapters and WHO guidelines for mental health in primary care).

CEBMH (Centre for Evidence Based Mental Health) (http:// www.cebmh.com/)

This organisation promotes and supports the teaching and practice of evidence-based mental health care. Information is provided to consumers about the centre's research activities, educational events and a gateway to various NHS websites on depression, schizophrenia and suicide as well as other high quality sources of mental health evidence.

NHS direct online (http://www.nhsdirect.nhs.uk)

This website provides high quality health information and advice for individuals within the UK. It is supported by a 24-hour nurse advice and information helpline providing details about various treatment methods available. The information is accessed from *Clinical Evidence*, the British Medical Journal's worldwide survey of the best and most up-to-date medical research.

Healthfinder (www.healthfinder.gov)

This website was developed for consumers in the USA. It provides those searching for information on specific health issues with material from a range of carefully selected websites posted by over 1,700 health-related organisations.

TRIP (Turning Research into Practice) (www.tripdatabase.com)

This is a meta-resource which provides access to high quality medical literature from a wide range of sources. The TRIP database's content is reviewed monthly and new material (approximately 300–400 new articles) from the publications covered is added to the site. The TRIP database is separated into a number of categories providing extensive material covering evidence-based information, clinical guidelines, query-answering services, medical images, e-textbooks, patient information leaflets and peer-reviewed journals.

Complaining about new media

To conclude, it is worth mentioning the avenues open to those who are dissatisfied by what they are accessing on the Internet. An important body concerned with complaints is the self-regulatory body the Internet Watch Foundation. This organisation works in partnership with the government, Internet Service Providers (ISP), telecommunication agencies and the police with regard to developing initiatives to minimise the availability of illegal content, such as child abuse images, available on the Internet. If the content is believed to be illegal, it can be reported to the self-regulatory body the Internet Watch Foundation. Illegal material includes that which contravenes national security, protection of minors, protection of human dignity, economic security, information security, protection of privacy, protection of reputation and intellectual property.

The message

Providing misinformation (quackery)

As already discussed, one of the main concerns regarding information accessed via the web relates to its questionable degree of accuracy or reliability. Kiley (1999) writes about this as 'Quackery on the web', relating to medical misinformation, and indicates the following categories: cure-all remedies, inaccurate information and biased information

Cure-all remedies

Many wild, misleading or inaccurate claims are made about health issues on the Internet. These are not always easily verifiable and may be hard to ignore especially for those desperately seeking information, support or treatment. One of the more disturbing trends includes the posting of miracle cures, inaccurate information and unverified claims as evidenced by Bower (1996) such as the acclamation of shark cartilage as a means of strengthening the body's immune system and inhibiting tumour growth and the development of cancer. While these claims may be instantly discredited by some users, others may be swayed by their level of desperation and anxiety about missing potentially life-saving treatments.

From a mental health perspective, a quick search of the Internet provides a range of impressive sounding as well as very dubious sounding remedies and treatments. Some of these are supported, in the absence of any empirical data, by a range of seemingly impressive claims and testimonials from satisfied customers. One site in particular, alternate-health, claims that a number of types of schizophrenia are caused by sugar-handling problems and that orthomolecular therapy can offer impressive rates of cure. Another site, vedicwisdom, states firmly that depression is caused by a fungus infection and goes on to say that it can be healed easily and permanently, urging people to send 105 dollars for two months supply of what essentially sounds like a foot balm. Naturally, no real evidence-base is given in support of the information that is offered in these examples with such assurance. Neither, in most cases are the credentials of the people providing this type of service identified. It is a shame that these points are not as easily determined by the site visitor as the ways in which payment can be made.

Inaccurate information

The problem with a number of Internet sites is the unverifiable nature of many of the claims being made, coupled with the delivery of misleading and potentially harmful information. This was highlighted in Culver, Gerr and Frumkin's (1997) investigation of Internet sites offering information about painful hand and arm conditions which found many providing misleading, unsubstantiated or inaccurate advice. Another area of concern relates to the increased range of material posted on the Internet by drug manufacturers, including a number of wild and unchecked claims about their products (Brannon 1999). Furthermore, a study by Lissman and Boehnlein (2001) reviewing the quality of Internet information about depression found that, overall, the quality of information posted was poor, with only half of the sites mentioning any diagnostic symptoms. They also found that half of the sites made no mention of medication, psychotherapy or professional consultation as suggested treatments for depression.

There may be an assumption that with the Internet we have a vast storehouse of knowledge, but it is clear that a lot of what we are exposed to can be regarded as misinformation. The problem is that those accessing the Internet infuse this technological medium with a greater sense of credibility than many other sources. When questioning this material, however, it becomes evident that it derives from every type of source imaginable, from the highly credible and verifiable to the overly subjective and unsupported. The knowledge accessed can only be judged reliable if it holds up against standard benchmarks. A significant proportion of the general public though do not have the ability or experience to discriminate effectively between good and poor information. It is particularly worrying where health information is being sought and inaccurate material is posted. Erbele *et al.* (2002) conducted a study to evaluate the reliability and validity of consumer drug-information sites on the Internet. They identified sites with an 'ask the pharmacist' option and found that fewer than 70 per cent of the sites answered the drug information question correctly, concluding that the information being communicated might be unreliable. Similarly, Bessel *et al.*'s (2003) study found that the overall quality of information provided by e-pharmacies on the Internet was poor. This is worrying news for consumers who are using the Internet as a means of empowering themselves and becoming more engaged and proactive with regard to caring for their own health, as they are exposed to material whose accuracy is hard for them to determine.

Biased information

A particular area of concern facing those searching the Internet for information about mental health issues relates to the degree to which they might be misled by biased information. This is where those posting material on the Internet have a vested interest in the message sent out, either for personal or commercial reasons, and as a consequence do not relate material from an objective point of view. As opinions and philosophies concerning the treatment of mental illness have for countless years invited fiercely opposing views it is hardly surprising that the range of information available on the Internet is so varied. It is like a market place where every type of viewpoint and perspective has representation although some are more prominent and better packaged. An example here relates to the sponsoring of Internet sites by pharmaceutical companies who offer financial incentives to organisations who otherwise would be unable to offer their information to consumers via this electronic resource. The extent to which posted information is geared to the needs of the sponsoring group clearly varies from the carrying of a brand mark or logo through to a more direct selling of the sponsor's product. Another example relates to companies that sponsor their sites with particular search engines thereby achieving a greater prominence. The first site that appears when entering the term 'manic depression' on the Altavista search engine is for an organisation selling a product entitled 'Serenity'. On this particular search there were 107,996 sites listed although these were preceded by a number of sponsored sites that included the one for Serenity. The site itself includes glittering praise for Dr Nieper, the product's creator and includes a number of testimonials from individuals who have used the product and who claim to have had their lives fully restored. There is no actual indication given though as to Dr Nieper's actual qualifications or experience to treat conditions such as manic depression. The site itself is very sales-oriented and includes many pictures of attractive smiling people. The ease with which this product can be purchased online and the lack of medical consultation means that customers are placed in the position of self-prescribing, swayed more by sales rhetoric than by an in-depth knowledge of mental health treatments. The examples listed above highlight the difficulty faced by the inexperienced or desperate person seeking the Internet for support. Distinguishing between the very varied messages and trying to extract what is most helpful seems a veritable minefield and individuals are therefore drawn towards those that are easily locatable and have glowing testimonials and effective-sounding credentials.

Searching the Internet

The issues discussed above highlight some of the problems facing the person using the Internet as an informational resource. Clearly, people have their own particular needs when searching the Internet for mental health information either perhaps as health care professionals or service-users. An illustration of the daunting and sometimes bewildering process facing the Internet user can be seen in the following example which considers a person seeking information after learning of a family member's diagnosis of schizophrenia. Obviously the initial instinct is to feel scared and shocked, wanting reassurance and information. There are a number of places we might go in order to find out about this condition such as to the GP, the library or the Internet. The first choice facing the Internet user concerns which of the many available search engines to use. If, for example, we type in the word 'schizophrenia', Altavista, Google and Yahoo all return over 5 million sites, whereas Ask Jeeves has 1,400,000 and Lycos only 680,000. The sheer scale of sites available makes it extremely unlikely that more than a fraction will be visited. We may, therefore, never reach those further down the list that potentially include valuable and helpful information which is therefore missed. Ideally the key is in knowing what to look for or having particular 'brand' names to try and locate. This includes the names of organisations such as Mind, Rethink or the Royal College of Psychiatry.

The service-user and professional groups are proving enormously helpful with regard to searching the Internet as they provide informative advice about various mental health conditions as well as links to related sites. This includes information about specific conditions, the various modes of treatment available as well as information about how to go about seeking help. A list of some of the core professional and service-user sites is included in Appendix 1. When assessing the quality of particular information sources there are certain aspects that need to be considered. A number of individuals such as Cooke (2001) have provided guides to assist in evaluating Internet sites. These are useful although perhaps need a few extra elements adding when specifically engaging with sites offering mental health content. These are provided in Appendix 2.

Suicide and the Internet

One subject in particular that has raised grave concerns regarding its coverage within the Internet is that of suicide. On the one hand there are many excellent, sensitive and informative sites such as those provided by the Samaritans and the BBC offering visitors practical advice and support in gaining help. These represent the responsible and better-regulated spheres of information obtainable. On the reverse side there are a number of poorly constructed, misleading, irresponsible and actively harmful bodies of information. This in part is due to the lack of regulation and means that very vulnerable individuals are able to access sites that actively encourage or instruct them in methods for self-harm and suicide (Alao *et al.* 1999). While some of these sites represent so-called pro-euthanasia organisations (e.g. the End of Life Choices, formerly the Hemlock society), others are posted by individuals whose motives are far from clear. The worst sites provide very graphically illustrative material such as copies of suicide notes, death certificates and colour photographs or, as in the case of the 'Church of Euthanasia', the inclusion of a telephone hotline with an A–Z of suicide techniques available. This disturbing picture is reflected by other sites that provide information on 'how to . . .', which relate to every conceivable method of suicide including hanging, electrocution or even snakebite. Product information via the Internet is also available in the book *Beyond Final Exit*, one of the many irresponsible resources obtainable. It is a book that is advertised with a fair amount of jargon and sanitising of terms, with 'self-deliverance' and 'departing drugs', for example, replacing the more stark terminology of 'suicide' and 'death'. It is advertised with classic 'sales-pitch' jargon attempting to make the product appear more desirable with phrases like; 'Common questions about poisonous plants – if you're optimistic about these, be warned of the side effects first!' These are appalling examples although, sadly, not isolated ones and they are perhaps surpassed by the availability of suicide kits (e.g. poison packs of potassium cyanide) that have reportedly been purchased from some Internet sites (BBC 2000). Just as alarming as this are the reported instances of suicide pacts that have been made over the Internet or individuals killing themselves online, apparently goaded by site visitors. The fact that these types of site are so freely accessible by confused and vulnerable people is a cause for grave concern (Thompson 1999). Andrew Solomon (2002), in his excellent account *The Noonday Demon*, aptly sums up the state of mind that people are experiencing when contemplating suicide. It reflects the sense of hopelessness experienced and the overriding feeling that others don't care, compounded by the fact that a person's capacity to recognise supportive gestures is restricted. The significance of this then relates to the type of views that vulnerable and desperate individuals are exposed to, whether it be supportive and containing helpful material, or uncaring and destructive. The worst types of site can for some seem very persuasive, reinforcing feelings of helplessness with the message that no salvation will be forthcoming and the only realistic option open to them is that of suicide. The overly pessimistic and negative rhetoric with which much of this material is presented might provide the only sense of acknowledgement and feeling of understanding from others that some individuals receive. These feelings of connection, although of a detrimental and unhelpful type, can prove extremely powerful in influencing vulnerable and desperate people or leading them towards certain actions. Those who are fortunate enough however to have located other resources such as the Samaritans' website will have a very different experience, with even the most desperate perhaps finding a degree of comfort and support from the feeling that others care and that various forms of help can be obtained. When accessing the Samaritans' homepage, visitors are initially greeted with the message:

> 'I was going through a really tough time last year. I didn't want to be a downer for my friends so I didn't talk to them. So I called the Samaritans. They gave me the time I needed. Now I can get on with my life.'

(Samaritans 2005)

This is complemented by a variety of easily accessible and navigable links that include details of how to contact them as well as information and audio examples about what to expect after calling. A new and important facility is now provided by the opportunity to use e-mail as a means of contact. What is important about the better type of site such as this one is the opportunity to feel acknowledged and supported by those who wish one well. It means being directed towards resources where a person can feel listened to and heard by others, considerably different to the sites that are more interested in presenting their own views or selling their products than in actually listening and showing concern for others. There are a number of implications here for health care providers including the need to be aware of the range of Internet resources accessible if they are to properly help those in extreme distress (Baume *et al.* 1998). This means directing individuals towards information that is supportive and emotionally containing, as well as helping them to express themselves and talk about the destructive material which they might also have come across. Because of the difficulties inherent in regulating or policing the Internet, these harmful and misleading sites continue to exist. Policing the Internet has resulted in various types of material, such as obscene and pornographic material, being barred or removed although it needs to be applied as strongly to material that encourages self-destructive behaviour. This should be aided by the creation of a greater range of sites that are supportively geared towards the topic of suicide prevention thereby combating the variety of poorly constructed ones (Mehlum 2000). One such example is the *Internet and Suicide Prevention* site, hosted by the suicide research and prevention unit at the University of Oslo in Norway. This organisation is dedicated to preventing suicidal behaviour, alleviating its effects and providing a forum for discussion between academics, mental health professionals, crisis workers, volunteers and suicide survivors. There are a number of other positive links obtainable through the professional and service-user organisations. An example includes the informative online booklet *How to Help Someone who is Feeling Suicidal* available from Mind's website (Mind 2004b). These resources provide a more positive outlook and will help to some degree meet the targets and recommendations for suicide reduction outlined by *The Health of the Nation* (DOH 1992), the governmental White Paper *Saving Lives: Our Healthier Nation* (DOH 1999a), the *National Suicide Prevention Strategy for England* (DOH 2002), the *National Service Framework for*

Mental Health (DOH 1999b) and the *National Confidential Inquiry into Homicides and Suicides: the Safety First Report* (DOH 2001).

Lastly, it is perhaps worth noting the pressure currently being brought to bear upon Internet companies to stop them hosting websites and chat-rooms that appear to encourage suicide. It is a move firmly backed by anti-suicide campaigners, mental health advocates and press agencies such as *The Yorkshire Post* (McGee and Whitehouse 2005). This is a welcome move that hopefully will begin to limit some of the most destructive and distressing material accessible online.

Online therapy

Building upon the rise in computer use a significant development over the past few years has been the availability of therapy over the Internet, aided in part by the current boom in e-mailing and text messaging that has heralded in an era of written electronic communication. The diversity and scope of what can be offered through this new medium is almost limitless and it seems that psychotherapy and counselling have not escaped its potential. It is a process that is referred to in a number of different ways and includes e-therapy, cybertherapy and online counselling.

Most of the better-designed sites make prominently clear to prospective clients that this type of therapy is inappropriate for anyone who is suicidal or has violent thoughts (Landau 2001). While this may be the case for online counselling there are plenty of sites 'selling' therapy through courses, work-shops or tapes without any reference being made concerning its suitability or any possible contraindications. Landau (2001) raises the ethical issues involved with online therapy, namely those involving a practitioner's training, credentials and licensing relating specifically to online work. Accessing a good site may appear a lottery to those without experience to recognise what so-called qualifications actually mean. The title of Dr, for instance, might be highlighted without any indication of a person's actual experience or speciality. This reflects Maheu and Barry's (2000) findings that there is a distinct lack of information about the qualifications of individuals offering mental health services via the Internet. Clearly, when credentials can be assured, those seeking therapy can choose with a greater sense of assurance that they may be helped, particularly as Lange *et al.*'s (2003) study showed that those who benefited most from online counselling and showed significant improvement were those who had accessed online therapists with recognised grounding and training in psychodynamic work.

There are a number of aspects that make online counselling an attractive option for both therapists and those using this service. Increasing waiting lists for face-to-face contact coupled with levels of urgency for help may make this an appealing alternative. Online counselling also proves attractive to many individuals who are physically unable to meet with mental health professionals or are in need of supplementary support outside of counselling sessions (Oravec 2000). It is a service therefore that can be offered to anyone with Internet access irrespective of location and most types of physical disability or illness.

A number of issues can be raised when comparing Internet therapy with face-to-face work. Cohen and Kerr (1998) found no difference in the effectiveness of computer mediated and face-to-face counselling when treating clients suffering from excessive anxiety. Detractors might point to the absence of many cues that aid the therapeutic process, notably non-verbal communication and the limited expression of affect. Alleman (2002), though, notes that emphasis can still be achieved via certain modes including the use of capital letters or exclamation marks. While this is true in the case of intentional forms of expression, it does not encompass the many aspects a person may be unaware of and are expressed unconsciously. There may also be a strong sense of incongruity between what a person expresses verbally or in writing and what is communicated through their body language. Online work therefore presents a number of barriers to understanding that can be picked up and worked upon in face-to-face contact. The type of engagement between therapist and client may be affected by a person's choice of therapeutic mode as illustrated by Alleman's (2002) findings that higher levels of personal information are disclosed sooner on a computer as opposed to during face-to-face work. While in some cases this might be advantageous it remains unclear as to the extent to which people who have disclosed too much too quickly might be left feeling overly vulnerable and exposed.

A matter of some concern regarding the offering of therapy over the Internet relates to the degree of security and privacy afforded (Oravec 2000; Campbell 1996). In response to this a number of major mental health organisations have issued ethical guidelines for online counselling including encryption and the identification of those having access to patient records. As well as protecting clients there are also issues relating to safeguarding the interests of the therapist, as there are no guarantees against their replies to clients being printed, circulated or published (Cohen and Kerr 1998). While a therapist's professional body or insurance company provides a certain level of security the need for caution in what is written is evident. This has implications with therapists feeling stifled because of concerns about potential litigation or being less expressive and spontaneous because of feeling overly aware about what they might be communicating. These considerations can have a profound impact upon the way in which the therapist–client relationship subsequently develops.

Offered alongside the range of one-to-one work available over the Internet are a range of self-help and support groups. These, according to Lamberg (2003), are proving attractive to people with depression and other mood disorders who are turning to Internet Support Groups (ISGs) as a safe place to bring their concerns. They allow patients to discuss the impact that their illness has on daily life, relate the experiences they have with clinicians and hospitals, share the benefits and drawbacks of particular treatments, review new research, as well as encourage people to seek help. The effectiveness of these types of therapeutic group is highlighted by Houston, Cooper and Ford (2002) who noted considerable benefits being identified by the participants. The main problems encountered were in finding the most appropriate ISG and the fact that some users were faking their disorders. Internet groups have also been found to be useful in suicide prevention (Mehlum 2000), especially for those who feel isolated and lack the necessary support in their available social networks. ISGs provide them with opportunities to ventilate their feelings and obtain help and containment from others.

As illustrated above there are a number of advantages and disadvantages offered by the online medium that will suit some while proving unattractive to others. It might also complement face-to-face work through offering a holding role for those waiting for available therapists or in providing an immediate crisis response service. A potential problem, however, is raised by Gold (1998), with some not choosing to seek out the necessary therapy or treatment needed while in the comfortable anonymity of cyberspace. Despite its limitations the Internet serves to widen the choice of what is on offer to those in need of psychological support with a number of types of services available. An interesting example of online support can be seen with the brief Internet consultations or 'web chats' offered by *Good Morning* television's Dr Hilary. These provide a type of live 'agony aunt' approach whereby individuals are offered consoling words and urged to seek further help. Opportunities for diagnosis are obviously severely limited through lack of face-to-face contact and only patchy symptomatic details are available. What this does offer, though, is a feeling of connection with others experiencing similar issues and an impetus to seek help. Even if the only benefit obtainable from this type of service is in helping people gain the confidence to seek help, then it is a worthy and necessary venture.

Anti-psychiatry sites

Although representing only one of a number of perspectives, the anti-psychiatry movement is worth mentioning here because of the potential significant impact upon those accessing various sites that argue against the use of traditional mental health treatments. Some of the anti-psychiatry sites strongly condemn conventional methods yet in many cases offer little or no viable alternatives. The language used is often persuasive or frightening, conjuring up images of *One Flew Over the Cuckoo's Nest* and the abusive and oppressive use of treatment. The Say No To Psychiatry site, for example, offers a very stark warning: 'All psychiatric treatments are harmful.' This precedes a long and rambling account warning others of the dangers and evils of psychiatric treatment yet lacking any real substance or direction. While we would hope that most individuals accessing this site would instantly note the complete absence of authorship details and overall absence of any clear arguments or alternatives being offered, it is possible that a number of individuals looking at this site might be swayed. This includes those who are already fearful of or disillusioned with traditional psychiatry, either because of the stigmatising way in which it is reported or a general lack of support or supervision demonstrated in their own experience of care. The problem is that the wild and fanciful sites that lack any real credibility undermine those that actually make valid claims against the misuse of psychiatry. The worst types are generally vitriolic and abusive of the mental health system, clearly representing the views of dissatisfied and disillusioned consumers. Their opinions, though, are not helpful to the multitude of individuals who can be aided and supported by some of the many good packages of care available. Although in general, questioning and challenging the care on offer can be seen as a productive pursuit, being influenced to avoid all practical help and being left to cope unaided with acute and distressing symptoms is not productive. For example, those accessing the site for the Antipsychiatric Coalition are greeted with the bold heading: 'Why psychiatric drugs are always bad'. The extra degree of stress provided by the word *always* indicates that there is no room for any alternative viewpoints. It is in massive contrast to the active encouragement of drug therapy for the treatment of manic depression posted by organisations such as the Manic Depressive Fellowship (a national user-led organisation and registered charity for people whose lives are affected by manic depression). It has to be mentioned that not all the anti-psychiatry sites reflect such degrees of unsubstantiated rhetoric although they do commonly argue against various modes of treatment. Commonly, no alternatives are offered which is a shame as the process of questioning and challenging the traditions of mental health care is not without its merits. A more balanced and considerate view can be found within many of the service-user sites such as Mind, Rethink, Sane or Together: Working for Wellbeing.

Accessing the Internet

The way in which information on the Internet is received is to a large extent determined by who is doing the searching. It is also affected by what the recipient is intending to get or the particular state of mind of those searching the Internet for information. For example, the stressed and overloaded health care professional or the desperate and suicidal person will not have much time to peruse the huge number of sites available. Locations that are hard to navigate around or those appearing further down a search engine's listed postings may consequently be disregarded. This makes a search of the Internet a bit of a lottery concerning those sites that are accessed and those that remain undiscovered. It also means that those searching the Internet are as likely to be directed towards supportive and informative locations as they are to misleading and potentially harmful ones. Although those searching the Internet come from a wide range of different categories and groupings, the categories focused on below are those of health care professionals and mental health service-users.

Mental health carers/professionals

It appears that mental health professionals are steadily embracing and engaging with new technologies despite Lukoff's (1999) concerns a few years ago that they were behind in learning Internet skills. Recent reports though are more encouraging highlighting the establishment of an increasingly 'mental health literate' community (Christensen and Griffiths 2003). The steady development and utilisation of new media resources while having much of value to offer also present problems in information overload, poor quality material, potential harm and lack of scientific evaluation (Christensen and Griffiths 2000). This in part is reflected by Scrivener's assertion that: 'The Internet is bringing a cornucopia of resources to our desktops. However it is simultaneously threatening to unleash an epidemic of information overload' (Scrivener 2002: 4). The problems with information overload are compounded by the configuration of many search tools that are programmed to retrieve as much as possible of the material available (Cooke 2001). The Internet is to all intents and purposes a maze, and it is very easy to become disoriented and lost. Indeed, the diverse range of sources and content concerning health care information highlights the need to establish the validity and currency of what is posted. As Hebda, Czar and Mascara (1998) argue, there is a need for health care professionals and lay consumers to evaluate online resources using the same criteria as applied to other sources of information. These include the credentials of the source, the accuracy of information accessed, the date of issue or revision, as well as the potential bias of the posting organisation or person. It is clearly impractical and disconcerting for the over-worked health care professional who has a limited amount of time and a seemingly infinite array of resources to consider. Scrivener (2002) identifies a number of the problems created through information overload including mistaking unrefined data for knowledge, using short cuts, stockpiling and failure to appraise information and time mismanagement.

Mistaking unrefined data for knowledge

Clearly when pressured and unable to sufficiently review the material accessed, some information may initially seem informative and appealing. On a more careful and detailed scrutiny certain questions or concerns might be raised about the absence of any clear evidence base for the knowledge provided. Unrefined, raw and unverifiable data may be taken on board by the over-loaded health care professional and disseminated as knowledge to colleagues and patients. This might then be received by others as reliable information because of the credentials of the person relaying the message to them.

Using short cuts

The taking of short cuts is influenced by the time constraints a person has to operate within, as experienced, for example, by the GP accessing material between consultations. As a consequence the most easily locatable sites will attract a larger number of visitors. Another consideration relates to which search tool is favoured by those searching the Internet as those offering fewer but more definite 'hits' might be preferred. This is also obviously affected by the abilities and experience of those searching the Internet and their knowledge of particular guidance available such as that provided by the National Institute for Clinical Excellence (NICE).

Stockpiling

This is another problematic feature where the pursuit and collection of data becomes an end in itself. Printouts and saved files fill numerous folders without much sense of purpose or opportunity for critical perusal and reflection. Obviously this problem is compounded by the amount of material that can also be stored electronically.

Failure to appraise information and time mismanagement

The ability to collect huge amounts of information and to store it may well outgrow a person's ability to critically appraise and disseminate it. This is particularly so in light of all the new information that is becoming available on a continuous basis. Therefore, before a person is able to review all previously stored material they will already have a new amount of information to sift through.

If we look at the above features and the already overstretched practitioners, it is interesting to look at how information is shared among the clinical team. Dawkins (1976) coined the term 'memes' to describe self-replicating patterns of information (or misinformation) that behave like viruses. Information is passed from one person to another gaining authority with each new person. This is in a sense a form of 'Chinese whispers' where a message progressively changes with each recitation. It is also the case with a number of Internet sites that recycle data and material from other sites and pass it on electronically with little evidence, in some cases, as to its original source. In a number of cases the authors themselves may believe in the authenticity of what they are posting because of their confidence in the Internet as a reliable source

Mental health service-users

The development of the Internet as an information resource has dramatically transformed the role of the health care recipient to one that is more empowered and informed. The reasons why service-users are choosing to use the Internet as an informational resource is illustrated by Brown (2002) as including:

- Seeking a second opinion
- More time to interrogate source
- Wide variety of resources available
- Dissatisfaction with traditional health care provider
- Convenient to user (continuous access 24 hours per day)
- Privacy, especially with embarrassing issues.

The points reflected here suggest that individuals are wishing to become more proactive within their care and better informed about the treatment options available to them as well. The Internet is regarded as a valuable and informative resource regarding a wide range of subject areas and a MORI poll conducted in February 2001 revealed that 60 per cent of people who accessed the Internet would use it to seek help for mental health problems. The fact that only a small proportion (9 per cent), believed that the information they were accessing might be unreliable suggests that for most people it is felt to be a trustworthy source. The attractiveness of this resource is aided by its convenience and accessibility as well as the degree of anonymity afforded. The continuous, 24-hour access to sites makes it a very user-friendly location from which to obtain information especially for those whose personal or work commitments makes accessing other places, such as libraries, a more problematic venture. The sense of anonymity is extremely important especially where topics or subjects sought after are potentially embarrassing or individuals are worried about the possible degree of stigma attached. If a family member has suffered a stroke or heart attack, for instance, it is generally felt easier to speak with others about this than it is if they are experiencing mental health problems. This makes the Internet and its available support networks an increasingly valuable resource. Information can be obtained instantly and easily from a multitude of sites without the initial concerns about how one might be judged or critically received by others.

Another advantage offered by the Internet is that of connectedness and a sense of *universality* The process of *universality* is a concept highlighted by Yalom (1995) – a sense or feeling of one's problems and experiences being shared by others. Therefore, through the Internet, an individual has the opportunity to feel part of a worldwide group, connected with others experiencing similar problems, and thereby feels less isolated. This is vital for a number of reasons as a sense of shame or stigma may prevent individuals from seeking assistance through other channels and the feeling of connectedness achieved through this electronic resource might provide the catalyst for seeking further help.

The ready accessibility of information on the Internet means that those in need of help are better informed and aware of the various forms of treatment on offer. It means that they can have a greater involvement with their care, acting more as participants than of passive recipients of care. The vast range of pharmaceutical information and services available on the Internet also allows individuals to self-prescribe from a certain range of products. To some, this is a positive move forwards enhancing the trend towards consumer empowerment (Dupuits 2002). A number of problems can be seen with this, though, as those accessing these types of services may not fully understand the implications of what they are presented with, being influenced by the sales pitch, biased and misleading information and impressive sounding credentials. A study by Graber and Weckmann (2002) looked at nine pharmaceutical company Internet sites as sources of information about antidepressant medications marketed by the company. All of the websites were found to contain information of an advertising and emotive nature. None of them indicated the cost of their products and there was scant mention of adverse effects. They concluded that the information presented was limited and that it was consequently difficult for prospective consumers to adequately compare products. These are worrying findings, especially for those who have opted to obtain medication over the Internet and who have been misled or only partially informed about these products. In some instances it might also mean that some are getting ineffective or harmful treatment and subsequently being denied products and services that would actually help them.

The caring relationship

The Internet has the potential to create the conditions necessary for transforming the patient–physician relationship to that of a real partnership involving shared decision making (Bauer 2002; Winker *et al.* 2000). One of the core aspects of this is the encouragement and development of patient empowerment and autonomy. Thede (1999) states that this brings a number of practice improvements as patients subsequently come to health care professionals with a more thorough understanding of their condition. The view of the empowered and informed patient is one that raises as many concerns perhaps as it does attractions. For a start we can consider the potential conflict to the patient–practitioner relationship where both parties disagree strongly as to the best course of treatment available. In some cases this might result in care being refused because the patient does not believe it to be in their best interests, a stance that might be based upon a reliable grounding or a set of erroneous messages obtained from the Internet. The degree to which patients are either informed or misinformed by the Internet presents a number of implications, therefore, for this relationship. There is also the issue to consider that almost every conceivable type of perspective is represented as mental health issues are offered through viewpoints as diverse as medical, psychological, social, religious or anti-psychiatry. While this is to be welcomed in many ways, there is also a large potential for confusion and misinformation. Patients may challenge treatment options on the grounds of misleading or conflicting information that has no reliable evidence base. There is also the issue of desperate individuals seizing upon every potential new treatment method posted on the Internet and finding them unavailable through their practitioners. An example of this concerns the reporting of a trialled treatment for multiple sclerosis using goat serum. It would no doubt prove distressing to read in the *Sunday Times* (25 January 2004) about the dramatic improvement in their condition of those taking part yet reading on the Multiple Sclerosis Society (MSS) website that the drug is not available to the general public. The MSS were more guarded in their claims stating that 'The strong anti-inflammatory component of the serum is thought by researchers to be "potentially useful" in the treatment of MS.' While the information brought by patients might be treated with some scepticism or rejected as lacking in scientific evidence it clearly alerts practitioners to also review these resources themselves for new and updated material. In this manner the practitioner and patient learn together and the person experiencing mental health problems is regarded as having something to offer. In some cases the patient will be better informed and more critically aware of their condition than the person charged with treating them. In others they might be hopelessly misinformed or exploited by some of the many poor sites available. The informed patient, though, is for a number of reasons welcomed by the health care professional who is already struggling with increasing caseloads, time constraints and limited resources. It can also, in some cases, limit the amount of time required for face-to-face consultations as patients can be directed towards various online resources. As well as the 'informed' patient it is worth considering the benefits brought by the 'informed' practitioner to the caring relationship. This can be seen within Galanter *et al.*'s (1998) online educational course in addiction psychiatry. They found that a large number of respondents were psychiatrists, the majority of whom indicated that it helped them understand a 'good deal' about the management of alcoholism.

Conclusion

The virtual explosion into the public sphere of new media technology has to a large extent revolutionised the communication potential of the media. The instant access to an almost limitless array of material is as exciting as it is daunting to the consumer. On the positive side, the availability of information concerning every conceivable viewpoint means that service-users and their families can feel more empowered and included within the process of care. It also means that practitioners can more easily update themselves on a regular basis. On a negative note, the lack of regulation and the proliferation of harmful and misleading material on the Internet continue to cause considerable concern. Of particular note is the difficulty that many consumers have in discerning between what is beneficial and what is detrimental to their well-being, particularly as the language and presentation of some of the worst sites appear to be deliberately geared towards the vulnerable, mistrustful or disillusioned (i.e. 'All psychiatric care is harmful and oppressive'). It is essential therefore that various initiatives are employed in order to tackle these problems including changes in regulation and a policing of the worst sites such as those that openly advocate suicide. This should be matched by the further promotion of the more productive and positive ones, as illustrated by the Samaritans' recent large billboard advertising initiative. The importance for health care practitioners is in being aware of the range of information available over the Internet which include the negative as well as the positive. Therefore, as well as being able to direct individuals towards the better sites (i.e. Mind or the Alzheimer's Society), practitioners are also aware of the potential range of harmful or misleading material that others might be exposed to. This helps health care professionals where necessary to begin to counteract and deal with some of the often very persuasive and harmful content that is so easily accessible, thereby enabling individuals to be directed towards getting the most supportive help for themselves.

10 And . . .

This book has looked in depth at the way in which attitudes and feelings about mental illness are influenced and shaped through the range of portrayals across a range of media sources. The resultant view is largely dependent upon a number of factors that include a person's prior experience and degree of knowledge with regard to mental health issues. It is also influenced by the potency of messages attached to various media products and the type of engagement an individual has with them. One of the main concerns relates to the types of message accessible and the sense of imbalance that is apparent with predominantly negative portrayals being found. The overly dramatic and sensational style of depiction found in many media examples has an insidious and unsettling effect upon those exposed to them and might be hard to shake off, even following access to educational and health promotional material. One of the core problems here is that mental health promotional material appears on the surface far less enticing or dramatically engaging compared to that which carries stigmatising or stereotypical content. Our reading of messages is therefore heavily influenced by negative depictions as accurate and realistic portrayals are undermined by the more familiar stereotypes that link mental illness with aspects such as violence or eccentric behaviour. In order to tackle this, initiatives or approaches are needed to challenge and restrict the range of negative products on offer and to replace them with a greater selection of realistic and accurate examples.

The ongoing proliferation of negative examples within the media indicates that regulatory mechanisms in place across the different media types are not really working. This can be seen in particular within the formats of television and the newsprint media which, despite being very tightly regulated as well as having clear guidelines (BSC 1998; ITC 2002; PCC 2004; NUJ 1999) denouncing the inclusion of stereotypical and stigmatising mental health content, are still regularly found to be acting against them. This is strongly influenced by commercial pressures that urge producers and editors on towards ever more dramatic and audience-pleasing depictions. The fact that many examples appear to go unchallenged is a particular cause for concern and can be seen as relating to either a lack of critical feedback or the relative ineffectiveness of the regulatory bodies concerned to bring about any change.

A glance at the Press Complaints Commission website illustrates this point as very few instances are noted where negative coverage of mental health issues has resulted in any consequent action being taken. One interesting example concerns a complaint made to the PCC about an article printed in the *Daily Star* on the 4 April 2000 carrying the headline 'Beast Chops out Jail Pals Liver'. It was subsequently followed by another article a day later headlined 'Mental Hospital Set Lector Fiend Free'. The complaint was made by the victim's sister concerning breaches of Clauses 5 (intrusion into grief and shock) and 1 (accuracy) of the *Code of Practice*. The complaint was upheld and the newspaper offered to print an apology and send some flowers to the complainant's mother although this was rejected. It is clear, however, that the number of complaints considered does not match the large number of examples that seem to openly flaunt the regulations as evidenced by items that are regularly found within the tabloid media. But it is also worth being reminded of instances when significant movement has been observed following the critical public receipt of certain media products, such as *The Sun* newspaper's sudden emergence as a mental health campaigner following the widespread criticism received for their poorly chosen coverage of Frank Bruno's hospitalisation for depression. This demonstrated the fact that mental health coverage could be handled in a more productive way if it was perceived to be in the best interests of those concerned to do so. It also illustrates the point that the overall picture concerning what mental illness is perceived to be can be influenced by a number of sources, particularly media personnel, health care professionals or service-user groups. The following section outlines briefly some of the core approaches being employed in an attempt to challenge negative opinion and work towards creating a better-informed and more caring public when it comes to the topic of mental illness. The three main areas being addressed are: connecting (*distancing*), educating (*entertaining*) and exposure (*exploitation*). These themes have been focused upon at different stages throughout this book and reflect the positive end of the spectrum, in sharp contrast to their negative counterparts that are included within the brackets.

Connecting

In order for attitudes and feelings about the mentally ill to alter fundamentally there needs to be a greater sense of caring and concern for their felt and lived experience. As has been seen in the case of individuals whom the public care about (e.g. Frank Bruno), the media can be forced to rescind their current stance and a level of informed debate and exposure can follow. There are many different types of portrayal that take the receiver into a close proximity with the topic or theme of mental illness. As suggested previously, this is not always a comfortable or pleasant process for the recipient as an unpleasant or uncomfortable state might be aroused. This is, on occasions, a deliberate effect as certain media providers seek to arouse strong feelings like fear or suspense for the purposes of entertainment. The value of connecting portrayals is that they allow receivers to catch glimpses of another's world, an experience that might appear strange and something they would not have been able to imagine or conceive of. It seems that the inner world of every conceivable illness type is able to find representation within the media as a whole although featured heavily within literature. This can be briefly illustrated by the following examples that cover a range of conditions including depression (*The Bell Jar, Prozac Diary*), psychosis (*I Never Promised you a Rose Garden, Briefing for a Descent into Hell*), Munchausen's syndrome by proxy (*Sickened*), dementia (*Out of Mind*) and alcoholism (*Under the Volcano*). The sense of connectedness is strongly employed by the use of techniques such as first-person narrative styles that take readers directly into the thought processes of those involved. It is also achieved with some potency within the visual media of film and television through scenes that illustrate something of the person's inner world. This is done by the utilisation of various approaches including narrative voice-overs illustrating to the recipient what a person might be thinking or feeling. An example here can be seen in the final scene of Hitchcock's *Psycho* where the audience is finally granted access to Norman Bates's disturbed and frightening inner world. Another approach is through the use of visual cues that allow observers to see what a person's hallucinatory content looks and feels like, as cleverly conveyed in the film *A Beautiful Mind*. These can be extraordinarily powerful experiences helping to generate a real sense of understanding and awareness as to what is actually being experienced by the individual with mental health problems.

A sense of connectedness with mental health issues is also aided through the process of identification. This incorporates Horton and Wohl's (1956) concept of *parasocial relations* whereby observers feel a sense of relationship and engagement with particular characters placed in front of them. Clearly, the type of connectedness established is influenced a great deal by the extent to which we actually like or admire characters being portrayed and relates strongly to the types of attitude subsequently developed. It is interesting therefore to note the types of characterisation that are most admired by audiences and include those that are kind and helpful, display positive social and non-verbal behaviours, are successful in coping with threats and are competent and resourceful (Hoffner 1991). It is sadly evident that these qualities are rarely applied to those depicted as having mental health problems who are instead commonly shown as ineffective, odd and menacing, in contrast to those who are seen as belonging to the 'normal' population. The importance of creating a wider range of likeable mentally ill representations relates to the enhanced level of concern that is thereby evoked for their welfare. It means helping to move the recipient away from the more familiar position of detached and unconcerned observer towards one that is more concerned and caring. Another significant feature concerns the range of qualities associated with a person in light of their perceived attractiveness. It is worth considering Hatfield and Sprecher's (1986) findings that physically attractive people are regarded as possessing more socially desirable personality traits than unattractive individuals. As the mentally ill have traditionally been portrayed as odd and unappealing, it makes a welcome change to note the wider selection of attractive characterisations that are currently being employed such as Judy Dench in the film *Iris* or Lisa in the television soap *Hollyoaks*. This provides audience members with more realistic and identifiable role models than the monstrous, strange and scary representations usually on offer. The concept of role model is an important one and prominent individuals who are universally liked can go a long way in facilitating a shift in entrenched or uninformed attitudes. The degree of desire that a person has to understand something of another's lived experience is important and this inclination can be seen as being generated by different types of catalyst. On the one hand this might be simply a means of satisfying morbid curiosity whereas, on the other, it might be that genuine and altruistic feelings are being acted upon. To a certain extent, these approaches are influenced by the type of mental health problem being experienced, differing significantly, for example, between neurotic and psychotic states. At the neurotic end of the spectrum, the response is more likely to be sympathetic, understanding and caring while the opposite pole, that of the psychotic representation, generates feelings of fear and hostility. This to a large extent is dependent upon the way in which these issues are portrayed, a difference that is starkly seen in the way stories are presented by the tabloid media. Depression, for example, is on occasions highlighted with words such as 'sad' appearing prominently in the headlines (e.g. 'Sad Kerry', a report about Kerry McFadden's experience of depression that appeared in *The Sun*). The word *'sad'* can be regarded from two perspectives, either drawing the reader into a sympathetic and concerned response or alternatively carrying implications of 'pathetic' and helpless. It is, though, in direct contrast to the way in which psychotic states are regularly covered with familiar stereotypical terms such as 'psycho' or 'nutter' being employed. The essence of this concerns the type of reaction being encouraged by the style of coverage which plays a large part in the type of response engaged in the recipient, be it sympathetic and caring or unconcerned and dismissive. The essence therefore of the connecting approach is of allowing those experiencing psychological difficulties to be better understood, leading to a greater sense of acceptance and inclusion by others.

Educating

Allied to the process of connecting with another's felt and lived experience is that of helping media consumers to appreciate the real facts about mental illness. This means providing recipients with accurate information as well as helping them to become more discerning and questioning regarding the authenticity of what they are exposed to. The need for clear and factual education is aptly illustrated by the many misleading and inaccurate portrayals of mental illness found in abundance across all media types. In order to combat this, a number of initiatives have been developed to help in the education of media providers as well as those accessing their products. This is aided through a number of major campaign initiatives targeted at tackling stigma and discrimination concerning mental health issues including the Mindout for Mental Health's Mindshift campaign, the Royal College of Psychiatry's Changing Minds: Every Family in the Land and Shift, a 5-year campaign run by the National Institute for Mental Health in England.

Because of the vast informational reach of the mass media, it is vital that those involved in communicating mental health messages are actually sending material out that is both accurate and realistic. It is important therefore to ensure that media personnel are updated and more fully aware about the content carried within their products. In order to achieve this, the development of good working relationships between media providers and mental health advocates is essential. In total it incorporates what can be seen as a tri-partite relationship (see Figure 10.1) with service-user, health care professional and media groups all working together. There are a number of benefits that can be gained through closer ties between these groups and that can result in the creation of products such as the *Guide for Journalists and Broadcasters Reporting on Schizophrenia*, a venture including consultation between the National Union of Journalists and the Royal College of Psychiatry. Liaison with the media is seen as a vital step in the fight against stigmatisation and discrimination by both professional and service-user groups. As a consequence, most of these groups actively train or advise their members about getting involved with media personnel. In a number of instances the result is a media product that reflects a sense of collaboration between those who understand mental health issues and those who understand the communicating power of a specific media source. An example is the Media Action Group for Mental Health, a West Midlands based group that puts together local stories for journalists reflecting a more honest and accurate and positive perspective on mental health.

Another approach relates to the educative potential that the media itself

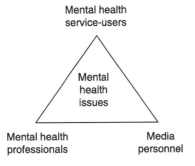

Figure 10.1 Media liaison and the tri-partite relationship.

has in helping individuals understand various aspects connected with mental illness. It includes projects or events that utilise examples from various media sources such as literature, film and music in order to enhance students' sensitivity to the personal experiences of psychiatric patients and to broaden their understanding of mental illness and the various methods used in its treatment (Wall and Rossen 2004). This is reflected in other successful studies by Frisch (2001), Bhugra (2003) and Hyler and Morre (1996) that employ cinematic examples as a means of developing students' awareness and understanding about specific mental health topics. The media with its multifaceted range of examples both positive and negative, historical and current, provides an enormous resource to dip into and examine the diversity of ways in which the topic of mental illness is represented. On a number of occasions the author of this book has devised and run a taught module (Mental Health Issues and the Media) that encourages students to examine the influence that particular mental health media messages have upon one's resultant attitudes. Student comments and evaluations have indicated significant shifts in approach with subsequent media engagement being carried out in a much more critical and questioning manner. One student in particular mentioned that she had initially been greatly amused and entertained by the film *Me, Myself and Irene* although on watching it again during the course of the module had a far greater appreciation as to how insensitive and offensive much of the content actually is.

Educating and changing a person's attitudinal approach is difficult and clearly does not rely upon information alone. Knowing that the majority of mentally ill people are not dangerous does not necessarily mean that we will feel safe and comfortable in the presence of those with mental health problems. One scheme in particular, the Mental Health Awareness in Action programme of educational workshops, was set up in west Kent schools in order to help tackle stigma and discrimination. It resulted in a significant change in attitude among those taking part and saw derogatory and stigmatising language being replaced by more sensitive and accepting words (Pinfold 2003). As illustrated by Haghighat (2001), one of the core elements in the success of workshops such as these concerns the opportunity for individuals to ventilate and share their anxieties and feelings. Many people need the opportunity to express and understand what their fears are actually based upon if they are to be properly able to accommodate and accept those with mental health problems.

Running alongside the presentation of clear and unambiguous material is the need to tackle and challenge the range of misinforming messages accessible. As already mentioned, these are plentiful and are strongly influenced by aspects of commercialism that encourage their continued appearance. As highlighted within a study by the Media Bureau (2001), the majority of journalists themselves observed that their reporting about mental health should be better. It is interesting to note that even those who are involved directly in producing stigmatising and stereotypical material would like to improve it but are swayed by pressures from other departments such as editors and production staff. It is therefore at all levels within media organisations that liaison needs to be developed.

A further approach concerns the provision of direct feedback to media providers regarding what is seen as either commendable or unacceptable coverage of mental health issues. This feedback is given in order to encourage the continued appearance of positive content as well as prompting media personnel to look at the potential harm that might be caused by poor reporting or inaccurate representations. Of course, some of the poorer styles of coverage are completely intentional and are unlikely to be swayed by persuasive arguments to the contrary. This is where the appropriate regulatory body can be engaged, with complaints directed to bodies such as Ofcom or the Press Complaints Commission (see Appendix 2 for fuller range of information). The importance of this is outlined by Philo (1996a) who states that those involved in creating media products should be more aware of the problems they are creating. Demands for change should not be left to mental health professionals but members of the public, service-users and their families should also be encouraged to get involved.

Exposure

Education and connection are both vital approaches although they are largely reliant upon the degree of exposure that various media products are able to achieve. As with the newsprint media, it is worth acknowledging the distinction between the tabloid and broadsheet styles, with the less accurate and more stigmatising format (tabloid) reaching a far more extensive audience. This is reflected across other media types where the dramatic and sensational is witnessed by a greater number of individuals. The challenge facing those involved with mental health promotion, therefore, relates to the uncomfortable fact that, for many, mental ill-health is far more exciting and appealing than mental well-health. The stereotypical and the stigmatising is the type of material that fascinates or shocks people and encourages them to buy into various products, enticed in part by the sense of dramatic content to be found within. Gaining maximum exposure for health promotional material means attending to the packaging of products and looking at the various ways in which audience appeal can be enhanced. In some cases this involves the offering up of products that are both entertaining and educative in order to get them noticed. This can be reflected in the effect achieved by some of the television dramas and soaps that combine somewhat unrealistic or overly dramatic material with opportunities to understand something of a person's experience. This is at times complemented by the provision of helplines and other contact details at the end of programmes for those interested in seeking support or needing to talk about issues raised.

The theoretical notions of perception and Gestalt theory have been addressed previously, focusing upon the attributes that help certain messages stand out from the background and be noticed. From a health promotional point of view, there is a strong need to investigate the particular character-istics of the channel selected for carrying a message. If, for example, the Internet is being used as a vehicle to transmit information, it is important to look at the various ways by which potential consumers are made aware of the existence of particular sites. This might be achieved through advertising or the range of content words entered when registering sites which are locatable through various search engines. The Samaritans organisation has helped to direct attention towards the existence of their electronic resources through advertising including a range of billboards carrying slogans such as: 'When was the last time anyone overheard an e-mail?' and 'The trouble with talking about things over the phone is the words don't always come out the way right' (Samaritans 2005).

Another factor helping to gain exposure for certain media products con-cerns the degree of intensity attached to content material. This can be achieved through the type of experience being recounted, as evidenced by the high popularity of autobiographical accounts dealing with appalling personal experiences such as child abuse or the murder of family members. Some of these accounts are linked to experiences that have already achieved a high level of exposure within the news media. They are ostensibly written as a means of putting the tragedy of personal experience into some sense of order and in gaining a degree of therapeutic value through the process of writing. There is also a significant degree of value on offer to others who have encountered related experiences and who are emboldened to share their feelings with others.

As has been seen above, the intensity of a mental health experience can cause it to stand out and gain greater attention. Maximum exposure is also achieved where particular psychological issues are associated or connected with individuals who themselves regularly gain widespread public attention. This can be seen where celebrities convey powerful messages to their audience, either of a self-destructive or of a self-nurturing kind. There is a long history, particularly within the music industry, of self-destructive behaviour being glamorised, even to some extent admired, and a person's tragic downfall helping to cement their iconic status, such as with Janis Joplin, Jim Morrison and Kurt Cobain. On a more refreshing note, there are a range of celebrities who are prepared to openly reveal and talk about their problems, allowing others to glimpse something of their vulnerable side. The current climate perhaps makes this a more accepted process than in previous years and includes a number of popular celebrities such as Geri Halliwell (bulimia/ depression) and Paul Gascoigne (alcoholism). The crucial message being sent out by these individuals is that of survival as well as the sense of optimism in that help is obtainable. Readers are hopefully emboldened by the courage taken to reveal what appear to be excruciatingly painful and embarrassing details. This process is aided and complemented by various initiatives such as the Mindout for Mental Health's (2001b) Headspace campaign whereby a number of music stars have spoken out about their own personal experiences of mental distress or that of people close to them. It can be illuminating and enlightening, therefore, for others to hear of the pain and distress that others have experienced and, in some cases, the identity of the person speaking out can be very surprising. It does help to demystify something about the nature of mental illness, certainly the fact that anybody, irrespective of background or social status, can experience psychological distress. This incorporates even those people who in the general public might pass off as having 'everything going for them' and therefore impervious to mental distress. It is a point raised by Geri Halliwell in her autobiographical account *Just for the Record*, stating how difficult it is to be met by such a misunderstanding attitude.

It is also worth mentioning here the exposure achieved by initiatives such as the World Federation for Mental Health's (2005) annual World Mental Health day, now being held each October as a means of publicising mental health issues and promoting better awareness among the general public.

Lastly, there is huge mileage to be gained in events that encourage and celebrate mental health expression and provide a sustained focus upon the topic of mental illness. This helps by gathering various products and modes of expression together and promoting them as a collective package, thereby gaining maximum exposure. An example of this can be seen with the Royal College of Psychiatry's Mind Odyssey programme of events that included multiple forms of expression such as film, art, dance, writing and music. This importantly provided both a means for creative expression as well as opportunities to question what those accessing these products were exposed to. Some of the films shown, for example, were followed by discussion panels (comprising health care personnel and service-user representatives) thereby providing a forum for exploration.

The way forward

The three issues identified above (connecting, educating and exposure) all help in the development of more adaptive images as well as looking at ways in which recipients engage with them. It is clear that the process of liaison is significant in helping to develop better relationships between mental health advocates and media personnel as well as enhancing the flow of communication between them. The maintenance and development of further health promotion/education initiatives will help in changing the 'total' picture of mental illness that is picked up by the receiver. It is this sense of the 'whole' that is important, as stigmatising and stereotypical depictions will never be completely eradicated owing to their attractiveness and commercial potential. The key, therefore, is in complementing the attention focused upon the media provider with a corresponding degree of attention upon the receiver. This means helping to develop the 'discerning' and 'interpretive' receiver as an individual who is able to thoughtfully question what it is they are exposed to. It might even represent the audience member who enjoys watching the film

Me, Myself and Irene yet is able to correctly distance Jim Carrey's facial contortions, exaggerated mannerisms and abusive behaviour with the 'collective group' regarded as experiencing mental health problems. It means partly starting the process of education at a young age, helping children to understand that the stereotypical characteristics they are exposed to are not representative of the 'total' group. Another aspect explored regards the process of perception and the type of 'filter' that messages might be passed through as a result of prior knowledge and experience. The space for people to express and make sense of what their fears and anxieties about the mentally ill are goes a long way in reducing the subsequent degree of discriminatory attitudes demonstrated as well as making people more receptive to factual information. Changing attitudes is not easy although certainly not impossible. If we relate back to Jastrow's duck and rabbit image (as seen in Figure 4.1) we can consider the issue that perhaps, for some, the duck is the stronger interpretation because it appears as a more exciting and attractive representation. Bringing another representation in front of the public's gaze is the main challenge although once we fully appreciate that there are two different interpretations we can move with greater ease between the two images. This, therefore, is the 'discerning' recipient, a person who is aware of the proximity of competing stimuli and is more thoughtful about the overall message taken away. The way forward for mental health campaigners is not a journey without difficulties although there have been some positive responses to various aspects that they should take heart from. If *The Sun* newspaper, for example, can be transformed, albeit very briefly, into a staunch mental health campaigner then one might believe that anything is possible.

Appendix 1 Internet sites – professional and service-user locations

Professional organisations

There are some very well constructed and clearly laid out sites aimed specifically at members of various professional bodies who deal with those with mental health problems. A selection of these is provided below:

Royal College of Psychiatrists (http://www.rcpsych.ac.uk/)
This site provides extensive material covering professional and practice issues. Information is offered about a wide range of mental health problems, various treatment options available and details of current initiatives such as the Changing Minds and Partners in Care campaigns. It also has links with published research, related articles and press releases. Specific information is also provided for professionals with regards to training courses or updating sessions available.

British Association of Social Workers (http://www.basw.co.uk/)
A range of articles, books and current news reports are accessible through this site. It also provides those accessing this site with links to other related sites. Professional advice and representation details are also given for its members.

British Association of Occupational Therapists (http://www.cot.co.uk/)
This site includes separately accessible material for its members and general members of the public who are directed to different home pages. A small range of mental health material is accessible via the 'public' site concerning legislation, treatment and certain conditions.

British Psychological Society (http://www.bps.org.uk/index.cfm)
This site is informative, is well laid out and very accessible. It has many links, press releases training and development, as well as information about finding a psychologist or making complaints. Careers and development, events and conferences, press and media releases, publications. Its accessibility is enhanced with the inclusion of a service for visually impaired users.

Royal College of Nursing (http://www.rcn.org.uk)
Some mental health information is provided although it is only accessible to members of the RCN. It includes the Mental Health Zone, which is billed as a one-stop shop for mental health nurses. This provides resources, policy initiatives, links and current news concerning mental health issues. Online journals, current news items, campaign initiatives and a discussion forum are also accessible.

Nursing and Midwifery Council (http://www.nmc-uk.org)
A range of research reports, legislative items and current news items are available through this site. It also includes specific professional advice for its members, various press release statements as well as links to related sites.

Mental health charities/user groups

Mind (http://www.mind.org.uk/)
The purpose of Mind is to challenge discrimination, influence mental health policy, as well as provide a voice and advance the views of those affected with mental health problems. Their Internet site is an informative location that offers a range of resources including online booklets, information sheets, newsroom items and details of policies and campaigns. It is easy to navigate around with good links provided.

***RETHINK* (formerly the National Schizophrenia Fellowship)**
(http://www.rethink.org/)
The aim of RETHINK is to help those affected by severe mental illness, including schizophrenia, to *recover* a better quality of life. Their site is uncluttered and provides a number of good resources such as the 'How mentally fit are you?' quiz as well as links and advice for other services (e.g. the Samaritans, 'contacting your GP'). Of particular interest within their main site is the @ease site, which is geared towards a younger readership encountering stress through issues such as exams, leaving home or starting work.

Samaritans (http://www.samaritans.org.uk/)
This is a well laid out and very inviting site including statements such as: 'It doesn't matter who you are – if you are in crisis, despairing or suicidal, it can make all the difference to talk about how you are feeling. You can speak in total confidence with one of our volunteers about anything that is troubling you. We will not judge you; we will not tell you what to do; but we will try to help you think things through. With Samaritans, you get the time and the space to find a way through.' It includes an audio clip resource that details what happens if you call.

Mentality (http://www.mentality.org.uk/)
Mentality is a national charity dedicated solely to the promotion of mental health. They work with the public and private sector, user and survivor groups and voluntary agencies to promote the mental health of individuals, families, organisations and communities. Their Internet site is an easy to access location providing a range of mental health promotional material, campaign information, news reports and related publications.

Sainsbury Centre for Mental Health (http://www.scmh.org.uk)
The Sainsbury Centre for Mental Health (SCMH) is a registered charity that aims to improve the quality of life for people with severe mental health problems. This organisation provides an excellent Internet resource that covers an extensive amount of information including practice issues, conference details, key discussion points, training material, as well as access to methods and tools for service review, evaluation and audit.

Maca (http://www.maca.org.uk/index.asp)
This is one of the country's leading national charities supporting people with mental health problems. They work in partnership with other organisations, such as primary care trusts and local authorities, to run a wide range of mental health services of which a good deal of material is provided on their website such as advocacy work, respite care and a range of therapeutic approaches. They also cover campaign information, current news items and have a range of downloadable publications.

Mental Health Foundation (http://www.mentalhealth.org.uk/)
The Mental Health Foundation bill themselves as the biggest website on mental health (and mental illness) in the UK. This claim is suitably reflected by the considerable amount of informative material and detailed resources concerning mental health issues available. They include information on problems, treatments as well as strategies for living with mental distress. This is complemented by related policy and published material, links with other sites and current news items.

Zito Trust (http://www.zitotrust.co.uk/)
The Zito Trust is a registered mental health charity seeking to highlight issues relating to mental illness and the care of those who are affected by it. They include information about treatment and prescribing issues as well as policy issues and inquiry reports. Their website includes some interesting resources such as a press office section, with access to press materials and an interview request mechanism for journalists to contact experts and patients with experience of schizophrenia.

SANE (http://www.sane.org.uk/)

SANE is one of the UK's leading charities concerned with improving the lives of everyone affected by mental illness. They include material concerning fund-raising and research, and have a discussion group facility as well as a section providing links to other related sites. An extensive selection of mental illness literature is available and they also interestingly include a selection of artwork painted by those with mental health problems.

Appendix 2 Evaluating Internet sites

The following provides a guide to those accessing various Internet sites as to the validity of the information posted. It relates specifically to sites carrying mental health material and the extent to which this either promotes or denigrates, informs or misleads, and is helpful or harmful. Prompts and areas for further consideration are provided by the text in italics.

Internet site
- What is the specific purpose of this site?
  (*Education, entertainment, campaigning or a selling of products*)
- Who is the targeted audience?
  (*Service-user, mental health professional or lay public*)
- How easily accessible is this source?
  (*Position on search engine list, links from other sites, published/advertised URL*)

Currency
- How up to date is the information provided?
  (*This can be weighed up against other sources. Are there any major omissions?*)
- Are dates provided indicating when the information has been posted?
  (*Home page, index or within the main body*)
- Is the information updated as new material becomes available?
  (*Some sites clearly list dates and provide site visitors with indications of this*)

Ownership
- Who has posted this information?
  (*e.g. Governmental agency, professional group, service-user organisation, media provider, pharmaceutical company or personal*)
- Is it a recognised organisation or group?
  (*e.g. Mind, Royal College of Psychiatry, Department of Health, BBC*)
- What are the credentials of those offering this site?
  (*e.g. Professional, personal experience, affiliation to user-carer group*)

- What possible bias could be present?
  (*e.g. Drug sponsorship or personal experience of care*)
- Have those posting information had any material published or presented elsewhere?
  (*Journal articles, books, official publications, television or radio programmes*)

Mental health promotion

- To what extent are mental health issues being positively promoted?
  (*Accurate and realistic messages, support and acceptance, campaigning*)
- To what extent could this material prove harmful?
  (*Inaccuracies, dissuasion re various treatment types*)
- Is any stereotypical or stigmatising content present?
  (*Imagery, terminology, overall content*)
- Does this site provide any links with other related sites?
  (*Range and quality*)

Presentation and site layout

- How easy is it to orientate around the site and retrieve information?
  (*Clarity of navigation, site maps, links to home page, index*)
- Is the information provided supported by any suitable evidence-base?
  (*e.g. Links to legislation and governmental acts, research material*)
- How accessible is the language used with regards the targeted audience?
  (*User-friendliness, jargonistic or technical terms, use by adolescent visitors*)

Appendix 3 Complaining about the media

Broadcast media

BBC
Tel: 08700 100222 (information line); e-mail: info@bbc.co.uk
Website: www.bbc.co.uk (includes contact details for specific producers)
Address: Head of Programme Complaints, BBC Broadcasting House, London W1A 1AA.

Channel 4
Tel: 020 73068333 (viewer enquiries); e-mail: righttoreply@channel4.co.uk
Website: www.channel4.com
Address: Channel 4 Television, 124 Horseferry Road, London SW1.

Channel 5
Tel: 08457 050505 (duty office); e-mail: customerservices@five.tv
Website: www.fivetv
Address: Duty Office, Channel 5 Broadcasting Ltd, 22 Long Acre, London WC2E 9LY.

ITV
Tel: 020 78438000 (programme complaints); e-mail: dutyoffice@itv.co.uk
Website: www.itv.co.uk
Address: Network Limited, 200 Gray's Inn Road, London WC1X 8HF.

Ofcom (The Office of Communications)
Tel: 0845 4563000; e-mail: contact@ofcom.org.uk
Website: www.ofcom.org.uk
Address: Ofcom, Riverside House, 2a Southwark Bridge Rd, London SE1 9HA.

The Internet

Internet Watch Foundation
Tel: 01223 237 700; e-mail: media@iwf.org.uk
Website: www.iwf.org.uk
Address: The Internet Watch Foundation, East View, 5 Coles Lane,
Oakington, Cambridge CB4 5BA.

Advertising (non broadcast)

Advertising Standards Authority
Tel: 020 7580555 (Complaints Department); e-mail: inquiries@asa.org.uk
Website: www.asa.org.uk (online complaints form)
Address: Advertising Standards Authority, 2 Torrington Place, London
WC1 7HW.

Newsprint media

Press Complaints Commission
Tel: 020 73533732; e-mail: pcc@pcc.org.uk
Website: www.pcc.org.uk
Address: Press Complaints Commission, 1 Salisbury Square, London
EC4 8JB.

National and local press
Complaints can either contact the editor of a particular newsprint title or
the journalist responsible for the story in question. Alternatively, correspondence can be sent to the letters page marked 'for publication'.

Advice for those wishing to make complaints

For advice or information about the style and content of complaints, e.g.
what to include and how to phrase it, the following are useful contacts:

Manic Depression Fellowship – www.mdf.org.uk (Tel: 020 77932600)
MediaWise – www.presswise.org.uk (Tel: 0117 941 5889)
Mental After Care Association – www.maca.org.uk (Tel: 020 74366194)
Mental Health Foundation – www.mentalhealth.org.uk (Tel: 020 78020300)
Mental Health Media – www.mhmedia.com (Tel: 020 77008171)
Mind – www.mind.org.uk (Tel: 020 85192122)
Rethink – www.rethink.org (Tel: 020 73309100)

Bibliography

Adams, T. (1998) *Addicted*. London: Collins Willow.

Alao, A., Yolles, J. and Armenta, W. (1999) Cybersuicide: The Internet and Suicide. *The American Journal of Psychiatry*, 156(11): 1836–1837.

Allan, S. (1999) *News Culture*. Buckingham: Open University Press.

Alleman, J. (2002) Online Counselling: The Internet and Mental Health Treatment. *Psychotherapy: Theory, Research, Practice, Training*, 39(2): 199–209.

Allen, R. (1995) *Projecting Illusion*. Cambridge: Cambridge University Press.

Alternate Health. *Schizophrenia*. Available at <http://www.alternate-health.com/schizo.html> (Accessed 12 March 2005).

Anderson, M. (2003) 'One Flew over the Psychiatric Unit': Mental Illness and the Media. *Journal of Psychiatric and Mental Health Nursing*, 10, 297–306.

Andreasen, N. (1987) Creativity and Mental Illness: Prevalence Rates in Writers and their First Degree Relatives. *American Journal of Psychiatry*, 144(10): 1288–1292.

Andrews, V. (1979) *Flowers in the Attic*. London: HarperCollins.

Angermeyer, M., Schulze, B. and Dietrich, S. (2003) Courtesy Stigma – a Focus Group Study of Relatives of Schizophrenia Patients. *Social Psychiatry and Psychiatric Epidemiology*, 38(10): 593–602.

Antipsychiatric Coalition. *The Antipsychiatry Coalition*. Available at <www.antipsychiatry.org> (Accessed 16 March 2005).

Appleby, L. and Wessely, S. (1988) Public Attitudes to Mental Illness: The Influence of the Hungerford Massacre. *Medicine, Science & the Law*, 28(4): 291–295.

Armes, R. (1994) *Action and Image – Dramatic Structure in Cinema*. Manchester: Manchester University Press.

Asch, S. (1961) Effects of Group Pressure upon the Modification and Distortion of Judgement. In Henle, M. (ed.) *Documents of Gestalt Theory*. Los Angeles: University of California Press.

ASH (2005) Available at <http://www.ash.org.uk/html/press/990528.html> (Accessed 22 March 2005).

Augoustinos, M. and Walker, I. (1995) *Social Cognition: an Integrated Introduction*. London: Sage.

Austin, L. and Husted, K. (1998) Cost Effectiveness of Television, Radio, and Print Media Programs for Public Mental Health Education. *Psychiatric Services*, 49(6): 808–811.

Bagdikian, B. (1997) *The Media Monopoly* (5th edn). Boston: Beacon Press.

Bagnall, N. (1993) *Newspaper Language*. Oxford: Focal Press.

Bandura, A. (1986) *Social Foundations of Thought and Action: a Social Cognitive Theory*. Englewood Cliffs: Prentice Hall.

Banks, I. (1984) *The Wasp Factory*. London: Abacus.

Barker, M. (2001) The Newson Report. In Barker, M. and Petley, J. *Ill Effects – the Media/Violence Debate* (2nd edn). London: Routledge, pp. 27–46.

Barker, M. and Petley, J. (2001) *Ill Effects – the Media/Violence Debate* (2nd edn). London: Routledge.

Barlow, S. (1996) *Heracles*. Warminster: Aris and Phillips.

Barthes, R. (1972) *Mythologies*. St Albans: Paladin.

Barton, R. (1976) *Institutional Neurosis* (3rd edn). Bristol: J Wright.

Barwise, P. and Ehrenberg, A. (1988) *Television and its Audience*. London: Sage.

Bauer, K. (2002) Using the Internet to Empower Patients and to Develop Partnerships with Clinicians. *World Hospitals & Health Services*, 38(2): 2–10.

Baume, P. Rolfe, A. and Clinton, M. (1998) Suicide on the Internet: a Focus for Nursing Intervention? *Australian and New Zealand Journal of Mental Health Nursing*, 7(4): 134–141

Becker, H. (1963) *Outsiders: Studies in the Sociology of Deviance*. New York: The Free Press.

Becker, H. (1964) *The Other Side: Perspectives on Deviance*. New York: The Free Press.

Belsey, A. (1998) Journalism and Ethics: Can they Co-exist? In Kieran, M. (ed.) *Media Ethics*. London: Routledge, pp.1–14.

Bennett, A. and Royle, N. (1999) *Introduction to Literature, Criticism and Theory*. (2nd edn). London: Prentice Hall.

Berlo, D. (1960) *The Process of Communication*. San Francisco: Reinhart Press.

Berlyne, D. (1960) *Conflict Arousal and Curiosity*. New York: McGraw Hill.

Berne, E. (1964) *Games People Play*. Middlesex: Penguin.

Bernlef, J. (1988) *Out of Mind*. London: Faber and Faber.

Berry, G. and Asamen, J. (1993) *Children and Television: Images in a Changing Sociocultural World*. London: Sage.

Bessell, T., Anderson, J., Silagy, C. Sansom, L. and Hiller, J. (2003) Surfing, Self-Medicating and Safety: Buying Non-Prescription and Complementary Medicines via the Internet. *Quality and Safety in Health Care*, 12(2): 88–92.

Bhugra, D. (2003) Teaching Psychiatry through Cinema. *Psychiatric Bulletin*, 27, 429–430.

Biocca, F. (1988) Opposing Conceptions of the Audience. In Anderson, J. (ed.) *Communication Yearbook*. Newbury Park: Sage, pp. 51–80.

Birney, E. (ed.) (1962) *Selected Poems of Malcolm Lowry*. San Francisco: City Lights Books.

Bloch, S. and Singh, B. (1997) *Understanding Troubled Minds: a Guide to Mental Illness and its Treatment*. Melbourne: Melbourne University Press.

Bloom, V. (1993) The Darker Forces: Freud and the Movies. *Journal of the American Academy of Psychoanalysis*, 21(1): 33–44.

Bobker, L. (1969) *Elements of Film*. New York: Harcourt, Brace and World Inc.

Bodenhausen, G. (1993) Emotion, Arousal and Stereotypic Judgement: a Heuristic Model of Affect and Stereotyping. In Mackie, D. and Hamilton, D. (eds) *Affect, Cognition and Stereotyping: Interactive Processes in Group Perception*. San Diego: Academic Press Inc., pp. 13–37.

Bolton, J. (2000) Mental Illness and the Media: the 13th Royal College Christmas Lecture for Young People. *Psychiatric Bulletin*, 24: 345–346.

Booth, A. (2002) Accessing Evidence-Based Practice. In McKenzie, B. (ed.) *Medicine and the Internet* (3rd edn.) Oxford: Oxford University Press, pp. 87–101

Borman, J. (2003) Depression in Women's Magazines. *Journal of the American Psychiatric Nurses Association*, 9(3): 71–76.

Borowski, T. (1959) *This Way for the Gas, Ladies and Gentlemen*. London: Penguin.

Borzekowski, D., Robinson, T. and Killen, J. (2000) Does the Camera add 10 pounds? Media Use, Perceived Importance of Appearance and Weight Concerns Among Teenage Girls. *Journal of Adolescent Health*, 26(1): 36–41.

Bourdieu, P. (1996) *On Television and Journalism*. London: Pluto Press.

Bower, H. (1996) Internet sees Growth in Unverified Health Claims. *British Medical Journal*, 313(7054): 381.

Bradbrook, M. (1974) *Malcolm Lowry*. Cambridge: Cambridge University Press.

Bragg, M. (2001) The Media and the Message. Edward Boyle Memorial Lecture 2001. University of Leeds.

Bragg, S. (2001) Just What the Doctors Ordered: Media Regulation, Education, and the 'Problem' of Media Violence. In Barker, M. and Petley, J. *Ill Effects – the Media/ Violence Debate* (2nd edn). London: Routledge. pp. 87–100.

Brannon, L. (1999) Regulating Drug Promotion on the Internet. *Food & Drug Law Journal*, 54(4): 599–621

Braudy, L. (2002) *The World in Frame – What we see in Films*. The University of Chicago Press: London.

Brindle, D. (2000) Ticking off at 11 O'clock. *The Guardian*. Wednesday, 4 October.

British Board of Film Classification (2000) *Sense and Sensibilities: Public Opinion & the BBFC guidelines*. BBFC September 2000.

British Board of Film Classification (2005) *BBFC*. Available at <http://www.bbfc. co.uk/> (Accessed 5 May 2005).

British Broadcasting Corporation (2000) *bbc.co.uk: HOME*. Available at <bbc.co.uk> (Accessed 6 September 2004).

British Broadcasting Corporation (2005) *BBC Guidelines*. Available at <http:// www.bbc.co.uk/guidelines/> (Accessed 20 July 2005).

British Film Institute (2005) *Screenonline*. Available at <http://www.screenonline. org.uk/film/id/790199/> (Accessed 16 May 2005).

British Psychological Association (2002) *Media Training Days*. Available at http:// www.bps.org.uk/about/bandc1.cfm (Accessed 14 May 2005).

Broadbent, D. (1958) *Perception and Communication*. London: Pergamon.

Broadcasting Standards Commission (BSC) (1998) *Broadcasting Standards Commission Codes of Guidance. Available* at http://www.bsc.org.uk/pdfs/research/ bsccode.pdf (Accessed 15 December 2002).

Brontë, C. (1983) *Jane Eyre*. London: Everyman.

Brook, R. (2003) *Mind Statement*. Available at <http://www.mind.org.uk/index.htm> (Accessed 24 September 2003).

Brown, H. (2002) Information for Patients. In McKenzie, B. (ed.) *Medicine and the Internet* (3rd edn.) Oxford: Oxford University Press, pp. 169–177

Brown, L. (2000) Entertainment in Our Extended World. In Valenti, F. *More than a Movie: Ethics in Entertainment*. Colorado: Westview Press, pp. 9–19.

Bruce, M. (1975) *Janet Frame: an Annotated Bibliography of Autobiography and Biography*. Wellington: National Library of New Zealand.

Byrne, P. (2001a) Imagining the Nineties: Mental Illness Stigma in Contemporary Cinema. Chapter 2, Part 4. *Every Family in the Land*. Available at http://www.stigma.org/ (Accessed 15 January 2005).

Byrne, P. (2001b) The Butler(s) DID it – Dissociative Identity Disorder in Cinema. *Medical Humanities*, 27(1): 26–29.

Calcutt, D. (1990) *Report of the Committee on Privacy and Related Matters*. London: HMSO.

Camp, D., Finlay, W. and Lyons, E. (2002) Is Low Self-Esteem an Inevitable Consequence of Stigma? An Example from Women with Chronic Mental Health Problems. *Social Science and Medicine*, 55(5): 823–834.

Campbell, L. (1996) How Secure is the Internet for Healthcare Applications? *Radiology Management*, 18(1): 28–32.

Carroll, N. (1996) *Theorizing the Moving Image*. Cambridge: Cambridge University Press.

Cash, T., Cash, D. and Butters, J. (1983) Mirror Mirror on the Wall . . .? Contrast Effectors and Self-Evaluations of Physical Attractiveness. *Personality and Social Psychology*, 9, 359–364.

Cassedy, P. and Cutliffe, J. (1998) Empathy, Students and the Problems of Genuineness. *Mental Health Practice*, 1(9): 28–33.

Chalaby, J. (1998) *The Invention of Journalism*. Basinsgstoke: Macmillan.

Chamberlain, M. and Thompson, P. (1998) Genre and Narrative in Life Stories. In Chamberlain, M. and Thompson, P. (eds) *Narrative and Genre*. London: Routledge, pp. 1–22.

Chan, J. (1993) *Wild Swans*. London: Flamingo.

Chatham, S. (1990) *Coming to Terms: the Rhetoric of Narrative in Fiction and Film*. Ithaca: Cornell University Press.

Chaudhuri, A. (2002) Why Weepy films are Good for You. Lifestyle Magazine, *Sunday Times*, 21 April.

Chibnall, S. (1981) The Production of Knowledge by Crime Reporters. In Cohen, S. and Young, J. (eds) *The Manufacture of News: Social Problem, Deviance and the Mass Media*. California: Sage, pp. 75–97.

Child, D. (2004) *Psychology and the Teacher* (7th edn). London: Continuum.

Christensen, H. and Griffiths, K. (2000) The Internet and Mental Health Literacy. *Australian & New Zealand Journal of Psychiatry*, 34(6): 975–979.

Christensen, H. and Griffiths, K. (2003) The Internet and Mental Health Practice. *Evidence Based Mental Health*, 6, 66–69.

Clare, A. (2001) Contemporary Images and the Future. Cinematic Portrayals of Psychiatrists. Chapter 2, Part 4. *Every Family in the Land: Understanding Prejudice and Discrimination against People with Mental Illness*. Available at <http://www.stigma.org/everyfamily/aclare.html> (Accessed 17 May 2005).

Clausse, R. (1968) The Mass Public at Grips with Mass Communication. *International Social Science Journal*, 20(4): 625–643.

Cohen, G. and Kerr, B. (1998) Computer-Mediated Counselling: an Empirical Study of a New Mental Health Treatment. *Computers in Human Services*, 15(4): 13–26.

Cohen, M. (1982) *Charles Horton Cooley and the Social Self in American Thought*. New York: Garland.

Collins, R. (1990) *Television – Policy and Culture*. London: Unwin Hyman.

Comstock, G., Chaffee, S., Katzman, N., McCombs, M. and Roberts, D. (1978) *Television and Human Behaviour*. New York: Columbia University Press.

Cooke, A. (2001) *A Guide to Finding Quality Information on the Internet: Selection and Evaluation Strategies* (2nd edn). London: Library Association Publishing.

Corrigan, P. and Penn, D, (1999) Lessons from Social Psychology on Discrediting Psychiatric Stigma. *American Psychologist*, 54, 765–776.

Cortazzi, M. (1993) *Narrative Analysis*. London: The Falmer Press.

Crepaz-Keay, D. (1996) A Sense of Perspective: the Media and the Boyd Inquiry. In Philo, G. (ed.) *Media and Mental Distress*. London: Longman, pp. 37–44.

Crisp, A., Gelder, M., Rix, S., Meltzer, H. and Rowlands, O. (2000) Stigmatisation of People with Mental Illnesses. *British Journal of Psychiatry*, 177, 4–7.

Croteau, D. and Hoynes, W. (2000) *Media Society: Industries, Images and Audiences* (2nd edn). London: Pine Forge Press.

Cuenca, O. (2002) Mass Media and Psychiatry. In Sartorius, N. and Gaebel, W. (eds) *Psychiatry in Society*. New York: Wiley and Sons, pp. 263–279.

Culver, J., Gerr, F. and Frumkin, H. (1997) Medical Information on the Internet: a Study of an Electronic Bulletin Board. *Journal of General Internal Medecine*, 12(8): 466–470.

Dawkins, R. (1976) *The Selfish Gene*. Oxford: Oxford University Press.

Day, D. and Page, S. (1986) Portrayal of Mental Illness in Canadian Newspapers. *Canadian Journal of Psychiatry*, 31(9): 813–817.

Deaver, J. (1994) *Praying for Sleep*. London: Coronet.

Department of Health (1990) *National Health Service and Community Care Act*. Available at <http://www.opsi.gov.uk/acts/acts1990/ukpga_19900019_en_1.htm> (Accessed 5 July 2005).

Department of Health (1992) *The Health of the Nation*. London: Department of Health.

Department of Health (1995) *Disability Discrimination Act*. Available at <www.direct.gov.uk> (Accessed 5 June 2005).

Department of Health (1999) *Safer Services: National Inquiry into Suicide and Homicide by People with Mental Illness*. London: Department of Health.

Department of Health (1999) *Saving Lives: Our Healthier Nation*. London: Department of Health.

Department of Health (1999) *National Service Framework for Mental Health. Standard One: Health Promotion*. London: Department of Health

Department of Health (2002) *National Suicide Prevention Strategy for England – Consultation Document*. London: Department of Health.

Department of Health (2004) *Draft Mental Health Bill*. Available at <http://www.dh.gov.uk/PolicyAndGuidance/HealthAndSocialCareTopics/MentalHealth/MentalHealthArticle/fs/en?CONTENT_ID=4089593&chk=t9P0rz> (Accessed 16 July 2005).

Department of Health/Rethink (1999) *Severe Mental Illness Explained – a Guide for Journalists*. London: Department of Health.

Devereaux, L. and Hillman, R. (eds) (1995) *Fields of Vision*. London: University of California Press.

Devereux, E. (2003) *Understanding the Media*. London: Sage.

Deveson, A. (1992) *Tell Me I'm Here*. London: Penguin.

Dictionary.com (2005) Available at <http://dictionary.reference.com/> (Accessed 19 July 2005).

Domino, G. (1983) Impact of the Film One Flew over the Cuckoo's Nest on Attitudes to Mental Illness. *Psychological Reports*, 53, 173–182.

Dupuits, F. (2002) The Effects of the Internet on Pharmaceutical Consumers and Providers. *Disease Management & Health Outcomes*, 10(11): 679–691.

Durkin, S. (2002) Predictors of Vulnerability to Reduced Body Image Satisfaction and Psychological Wellbeing in Response to Exposure to Idealized Female Media Images in Adolescent Girls. *Journal of Psychosomatic Research*, 53(5): 995–1005.

Easton-Ellis, B. (1991) *American Psycho*. Basingstoke: Picador.

Eco, U. (1989) *The Open Work*. London: Hutchinson.

Elliott, J. (2005) *The Little Prisoner*. London: Harper Element.

Epting, F. (1984) *Personal Construct Counselling and Psychotherapy*. Chichester: John Wiley.

Erbele, S., Riggins, J., Williams, C. and Heck, A. (2002) Evaluating Internet Drug Information. *Hospital Pharmacy*, 37(2): 141–145.

European Information Society Group. (2004) *Current Internet Regulation Issues*. Available at <http://www.eurim.org/briefings/IWF_eurim2.htm> (Accessed 8 February 2005).

European Union (2001) *Television Without Frontiers Directive*. Available at <http://www.dentonwildesapte.com/assets/T/TVWithoutFrontiersDirective_Nov2001.pdf> (Accessed 21 July 2005).

Evans, E., Rutberg, J., Sather, C. and Turner, C. (1991) Content Analysis of Contemporary Teen Magazines for Adolescent Females. *Youth and Society*, 23(1): 99–120.

Feder, L. (1980) *Madness in Literature*. Princeton: Princeton University Press.

Ferrier, C. (1995) *The Janet Frame Reader*. London: Women's Press.

Feshbach, N. and Feshbach, S. (1997) Children's Empathy and the Media: Realizing the Potential of Television. In Kirschner, S. and Kirschner, D. (eds) *Perspectives on Psychology and the Media*. Washington: American Psychological Association, pp. 3–27.

Feshbach, S. and Singer, R. (1971) *Television and Aggression: an Experimental Field Theory*. San Francisco: Jossey Bass.

Film Education (2005) *Film Education*. Available at <http://www.filmeducation.org/secondary/concept/film-real/docs/real6.html> (Accessed 16 May 2005).

Fiske, J. and Hartley, J. (1978) *Reading Television*. London: Routledge.

Fitch, J. (1999) *White Oleander*. London: Virago Press.

Flemming, M. and Manvell, R. (1985) *Images of Madness: The Portrayal of Insanity in the Feature Film*. Cranbury NJ: Associated University Press.

Flemming, M. and Manvell, R. (1994) Through a Lens Darkly. In Rieger, B. (ed.) *Dionysus in Literature: Essays in Madness*, pp. 49–57.

Foucault, M. (1961) *Madness and Civilisation*. London: Routledge.

Foucault, M. (1979) What is an Author? In Harari, J. (ed.) *Textual Strategies: Perspectives in Post Structuralist Criticism*. London: Methuen, pp. 145–148.

Frame, J. (1961) *Faces in the Water*. London: The Women's Press.

Frame, J. (1980) *Scented Gardens for the Blind*. London: The Women's Press.

Frame, J. (1984) *An Angel at my Table*. London: Paladin.

Frame, J. (2002) *Owls do Cry*. London: The Women's Press.

Francis, C., Pirkis, J., Blood, R., Dunt, D., Burgess, P., Morley, B., Stewart, A. and Putnis, P. (2004) The Portrayal of Mental Health and Illness in Australian Non-Fiction Media. *Australian and New Zealand Journal of Psychiatry*, 38(7): 541–546.

Frisch, L. (2001) Friday Night at the Movies. In Frisch, N. and Frisch, L. (eds) *Psychiatric Mental Health Nursing*. Albany, NY: Delmar Publishers, pp. 779–799.

Frith, S. (1986) Hearing Secret Harmonies. In McCabe, C. (ed.) *High Theory/Low Culture: Analysing Popular Television and Film.* Manchester: Manchester University Press, pp. 53–70.

Gabbard, G. (2001) Psychotherapy in Hollywood Cinema. *Australasian Psychiatry,* 9(4): 365–369.

Gabbard, G. and Gabbard, K. (1992) Cinematic Stereotypes Contributing to the Stigmatisation of Psychiatrists. In Fink, P. and Tasman, A. *Stigma and Mental Illness.* Washington, DC: American Psychiatric Press, pp. 113–126.

Gabbard, G. and Gabbard, K. (1999) *Psychiatry and the Cinema* (2nd edn). London: American Psychiatric Press.

Galanter, M., Keller, D., Dermatis, H. and Biderman, D. (1998) Use of the Internet for Addiction Education. Combining Network Therapy with Pharmacotherapy. *American Journal on Addictions,* 7(1): 7–13.

Gascoigne, P. (2005) *Gazza: My Story.* London: Headline Book Publishing.

Gauntlett, D. (1995) *Moving Experiences.* London: John Libbey.

Gauntlett, D. (2001) The Worrying Influence of Media Effects Studies. In Barker, M. and Petley, J. *Ill Effects – the Media/Violence Debate* (2nd edn). London: Routledge, pp. 47–62.

Gauntlett, D. and Hill, A. (1999) *TV Living: Television, Culture and Everyday Life.* London: Routledge.

Genette, G. (1980) *Narrative Discourse.* Oxford: Blackwell.

Geraghty, C. (1991) *Women and Soap Opera.* Cambridge: Polity Press.

Gilbert, P. (2003) Shame, Stigma and the Family: 'Skeletons in the Cupboard' and the Role of Shame. In Crisp, A. *Every Family in the Land: Understanding prejudice and discrimination against people with mental illness.* Available at <http://www.stigma.org/> (Accessed 6 May 2005).

Gladstein, G. (1983) Understanding Empathy. Integrating Counselling, Developmental and Social Psychology Perspectives. *Journal of Counselling Psychology,* 30(4): 467–482.

GMTV (2004) *Dr Hilary's Web Chats.* Available at <http://www.gmtv.co.uk/index.cfm?articleid=2144&pageNumber=2> (Accessed 9 September 2004).

Goffman, E. (1961) *Asylums.* Middlesex: Pelican.

Goffman, E. (1963) *Stigma: Notes on Management of Spoiled Identity.* Harmondsworth: Penguin.

Goffman, E. (1974) *Frame Analysis.* London: Penguin.

Gold, J. (1998) Mental Health and the Internet. *Computers in Nursing,* 16(2): 85–6, 89.

Graber, M. and Weckmann, M. (2002) Pharmaceutical Company Internet Sites as Sources of Information about Antidepressant Medications. *CNS Drugs,* 16(6): 419–423

Grace, S. (1982) *The Voyage That Never Ends.* Vancouver: University of British Columbia Press.

Graham, G. (1999) *The Internet: a Philosophical Inquiry.* London: Routledge.

Gray, A. (2002) Stigma in Psychiatry. *Journal of the Royal Society of Medicine,* 95(2): 72–76.

Grazia, E. and Newman, R. (1982) *Banned Films.* London: R. R. Bowker.

Green, H. (1964) *I Never Promised You a Rose Garden.* London: Pan.

Greenberg, H. and Gabbard, K. (1990) *Reel Signification: an Anatomy of Psychoanalytic Film Criticism,* 77(1): 89–110.

Gregory, J. (2003) *Sickened.* London: Arrow.

Gripsrud, J. (2002) *Understanding Media Culture*. London: Arnold.

Gunter, B. (1987) *Poor Reception*. Hillsdale NJ: Lawrence Erlbaum.

Gunter, B. and Wober, M. (1992) *The Reactive Viewer: a Review of Research on Audience Reaction Measurement*. London: John Libbey.

Haghighat, R. (2001) A Unitary Theory of Stigmatisation. *British Journal of Psychiatry*, 178, 207–215.

Hall, S. (1974a) *Encoding and Decoding in the Television Discourse*. Centre for Contemporary Cultural Studies, Stencilled Occasional Paper No. 7. Birmingham: University of Birmingham.

Hall, S. (1974b) The Television Discourse: Encoding and Decoding. *Education and Culture*, 25, 8–14.

Hall, S. (1981) The Determinations of News Photographs. In Cohen, S. and Young, J. (eds) *The Manufacture of News*. London: Constable, pp. 226–243.

Hall, S., Critcher, S., Jefferson, T., Clarke, J. and Roberts, B. (1978) *Policing the Crisis*. London: Macmillan.

Hallam, A. (2002) Media Influences on Mental Health Policy: Long Term Effects of the Clunis and Silcock Cases. *International Review of Psychiatry*, 14(1): 26–33.

Halliwell, G. (2003) *Just For the Record*. London: Ebury Press.

Hamilton, K. and Waller, G. (1993) Media Influences of Body Size Estimation in Anorexia and Bulimia: an Experimental Study. *British Journal of Psychiatry*, 162, 837–840.

Hamlyn, D. (1957) *The Psychology of Perception: a Philosophical Examination of Gestalt Theory and Derivative Theories of Perception*. London: Routledge and Kegan Paul.

Haney, C. and Zimbardo, P. (1998) The Past and Future of U.S. Prison Policy: Twenty Five Years after the Stanford Prison Experiment. *American Psychologist*, 53(7): 709–727.

Hannah, D. (1978) Faces In the Water: Case History or Work of Fiction? In Delbaere, J. (ed.) *Bird, Hawk, Bogie: Essays on Janet Frame*. Denmark: Dangaroo Press, pp. 45–52.

Harris, C. and Lester, P. (2002) *Visual Journalism: a Guide for New Media Professionals*. London: Allyn and Bacon.

Harrison, G., Owens, D., Holton, A., Neilson, D. and Boot, D. (1988) A Prospective Study of Severe Mental Disorder in Afro-Caribbean Patients. *Psychological Medicine*, 11, 289–302.

Hatfield, E. and Sprecher, S. (1986) *Mirror, Mirror . . . The Importance of Looks in Everyday Life*. New York: State University of New York Press.

Hawes, C. (1996) *Mania and Literary Style*. Cambridge: Cambridge University Press.

Hawton, K., Simkin, S., Deeks, J., O'Connor, S., Keen, A., Altman, D., Philo, G. and Bulstrode, C. (1999) Effects of a Drug Overdose in a Television Drama on Presentations to Hospital for Self Poisoning: Time Series and Questionnaire Study. *British Medical Journal*, 318, 972–977.

Hayden, T. (2004) *One Child*. London: Element Books.

Health Education Authority (1997) *Mental Health and the National Press*. London: Health Education Authority.

Health Education Authority (1999) *Media Mentality: How the Print and Broadcast Media Treat Mental Health Issues*. London: Health Education Authority.

Health on the Net. *Honcode*. Available at <http://www.hon.ch/> (Accessed 22 July 2005).

Hebda, T., Czar, P. and Mascara, C. (1998) *Handbook of Informatics for Nurses and Health Care Professionals.* Reading: Addison Wesley.

Heller, J. (1961) *Catch 22.* London: Vintage.

Henderson, L. (1996) Selling Suffering: Mental Illness and Media Values. In Philo, G. (ed.) *Media and Mental Distress.* London: Longman, pp. 18–36.

Hersch, W. Gorman, P. and Sacharek, L. (1998) Applicability and Quality of Information for Answering Clinical Questions on the Web. *Journal of the American Medical Association,* 280(15): 1244–1245.

Hershkowitz, D. (1998) *The Madness of Epic.* Oxford: Clarendon Press.

Hesse, H. (2001) *Steppenwolf.* London: Penguin.

Hetherington, A. (1985) *News, Newspapers and Television.* London: Macmillan.

Hobson, D. (1988) *Crossroads. The Drama of a Soap Opera.* London: Methuen.

Hodgkinson, J. (1986) Disney's Return to Oz, and ECT. *Biological Psychiatry,* 21(5–6): 578.

Hoffner, C. and Cantor, J. (1991) Perceiving and Responding to Mass Media Characters. In Bryant, J. and Zillman, D. (eds) *Responding to the Screen: Reception and Reaction Process.* New Jersey: Lawrence Erlbaum, pp. 63–101.

Höijer, B. (1998) Social Psychological Perspectives in Reception Analysis. In Dickinson, R., Harindranath, R. and Linné, O. (eds) *Approaches to Audiences.* London: Arnold, pp. 166–183.

Holland, N. (1980) Unity Identity Text Self. In Tompkins, J. (ed.) *Reader-Response Criticism From Formalism to Post Structuralism.* Baltimore: John Hopkins University Press. pp. 118–133.

Horton, D. and Wohl, R. (1956) Mass Communication and Para-Social Interaction. *Psychiatry,* 19, 215–229.

House of Commons (2001) *Culture, Media and Sport – Second Report (7 March 2001)* Available at <http://www.parliament.the-stationery-office.co.uk/pa/cm200001/cmselect/cmcumeds/161/16108.htm> (Accessed 14 June 2005).

Houston, T., Cooper, L. and Ford, D. (2002) Internet Support Groups for Depression: A 1- Year Prospective Cohort Study. *American Journal of Psychiatry,* 159(12): 2062–2068.

Howlett, M. (1998) *Medication, Non-Compliance and Mentally Disordered Offenders: The Role of Non-Compliance in Homicide by People with Mental Illness and Proposals for Future Policy.* London: The Zito Trust.

Hughes, T. (1985) Ariel Ascending. In Alexander, P. (ed.) *Sylvia Plath and her Journals.* New York: Harper and Row, pp. 153–154.

Hyler, S. and Morre, J. (1996) Teaching Psychiatry? Let Hollywood Help! Suicide in the Cinema. *Academic Psychiatry,* 20(4): 212–219.

Independent Television Commission (2002) *The ITC Programme Code January 2002.* Available at <http://www.ITC.co.uk> (Accessed 12 December 2002).

Ingram, A. (1991) *The Madhouse of Language: Writing and Reading Madness in the Eighteenth Century.* London: Routledge.

Internet Service Providers Association. *ISPA.* Available at <http://www.ispa.org.uk/html/index3.html?frame=http%3A//www.ispa.org.uk/html/about_ispa/index.html> (Accessed 14 June 2005).

Internet Watch Foundation. *IWF.* Available at <www.iwf.org.uk> (Accessed 23 May 2005).

Jackson, P., Stevenson, N. and Brooks, K. (2001) *Making Sense of Men's Magazines. Men's Health Magazines.* Cambridge: Polity Press.

Jadad, A. and Gagliardi, A. (1998) Rating Health Information on the Internet; Navigating to Knowledge or to Babel. *Journal of the American Medical Association*, 279(8): 611–614.

Jamison, K. (1989) Mood Disorders and Patterns of Creativity in British Writers and Artists. *Psychiatry*, 52(2): 125–134.

Jamison, K. (1993) *Touched with Fire: Manic Depression and the Artistic Temperament.* New York: The Free Press.

Jamison, K. (1996) Mood Disorders, Creativity and the Artistic Temperament. In Schildkraut, J. and Otero, A. (eds) *Depression and the Spiritual in Modern Art: Homage to Miro.* Oxford: John Wiley, pp. 15–32.

Jamison, K. (1997) *An Unquiet Mind: Memoirs of Moods and Madness.* London: Picador.

Jensen, K. (1988) News as a Social Resource. *European Journal of Communication*, 3(3): 275–301.

Jinks, G. (2000) Therapeutic Skills and Clinical Practice. In Feltham, C. and Horton, I. (eds) *Handbook of Counselling and Psychotherapy.* London: Sage, pp. 122–151.

Johnson-Cartee, K. (2005) *News, Narratives and News Framing.* Oxford: Rowman and Littlefield.

Johnstone, M. (2001) Stigma, Social justice and the Rights of the Mentally Ill: Challenging the Status Quo. *Australian, New Zealand Journal of Mental Health Nursing*, 10(4): 200–209.

Kafka, F. (1933) *Metamorphosis and Other Stories.* London: Penguin.

Kalbfleisch, P. (1979) *The Portrayal of the Killer in Society: A Comparison Study.* PhD Dissertation. Department of Communication, Michigan State University.

Kanouse, D. and Hanson, L. (1972) Negativity in Evaluations. In Jones, E., Kanouse, D., Kelley, H., Nisbett, R., Valins, S. and Weiner, B. (eds) *Attribution: Perceiving the Causes of Behaviour.* Morristown, NJ: General Learning Press, pp. 1–16.

Kantor, D. and Gelineau, V. (1965) Social Processes in Support of Chronic Deviance. *International Journal of Social Psychiatry*, 11, 280–289.

Kent, R. (1994) Measuring Media Audiences: the Way Ahead. In Kent, R. (ed.) *Measuring Media Audiences.* London: Routledge.

Kesey, K. (1962) *One Flew over the Cuckoo's Nest.* London: Picador.

Kiley, R. (1999) *Medical Information on the Internet: a Guide for Health Professionals* (2nd edn). Edinburgh: Churchill Livingstone.

King, D. and Wertheimer, M. (2005) *Max Wertheimer and Gestalt Theory.* London: Transaction.

Kirschenbaum, H. and Henderson, V. (eds) (1990) *Carl Rogers: Dialogues: Conversations with Martin Buber, Paul Tillich, B.F. Skinner, Gregory Bateson, Michael Polanyi, Rollo May, and Others.* London: Constable.

Kitwood, T. (1997) *Dementia Reconsidered: the Person Comes First.* Buckingham: Open University Press.

Kitzinger, J. (1999) A Sociology of Media Power: Key Issues in Audience Reception Research. In Philo, G. (ed.) *Message Received.* Harlow: Addison Wesley Longman, pp. 3–20

Köhler, W. (1929) *Gestalt Psychology.* New York: H. Liveright.

Köhler, W. (1947) *Gestalt Psychology – an Introduction to New Concepts in Modern Psychology.* London: New English Library.

Kolker, R. (1988) *A Cinema of Loneliness* (2nd edn). Oxford: Oxford University Press.

Kress, G. and Leeuwen, T. (1998) Front Pages: (The Critical) Analysis. In Bell, A. and Garrett, P. (eds) *Approaches to Media Discourse*. Oxford: Blackwell, pp. 186–219.

LaBruzza, A. (1997) *The Essential Internet: a Guide for Psychotherapists and other Mental Health Professionals*. London: Jason Aronson.

Laing, R. (1990) *The Divided Self: an Existential Study in Sanity and Madness*. Harmondsworth: Penguin.

Lamb, W. (2000) *I Know This Much is True*. London: HarperCollins.

Lamberg, L. (2003) Online Empathy for Mood Disorders: Patients Turn to Internet Support Groups. *Journal of the American Medical Association*, 289(23): 3073–3077.

Landau, B. (2001) Psychotherapy Online in 2001: For Psychotherapists new to the Internet. *Journal of Mental Imagery*, 25(1–2): 65–82.

Landesman, C. (2005) The Sea Inside. *Sunday Times Culture Magazine*, 13 February, p. 19.

Lange, A., Rietdijk, D., Hudcovicova, M. van de Ven, J., Schrieken, B. and Emmelkamp, P. (2003) Interapy: A Controlled Randomised Trial of the Standard-ized Treatment of Posttraumatic Stress through the Internet. *Journal of Consulting and Clinical Psychology*, 71(5): 901–909.

Laurance, J. (2003) *Pure Madness: How Fear Drives the Mental Health System*. London: Routledge.

Lauronen, E., Veijola, J, Isohanni, I., Jones, P., Nieminem, P. and Isohanni, M. (2004) Links Between Creativity and Mental Disorder. *Psychiatry*, 67(1): 81–98.

Lawrence, D.H. (1972) *Lady Chatterley's Lover*. New York: Viking Press.

Lee, C. (2005) *To Die For*. London: Arrow.

Lessing, D. (1971) *Briefing for a Descent into Hell*. St Albans: Panther.

Link, B., Struening, E., Neese-Todd, S., Asmussen, S. and Phelan, J. (2001) The Consequences of Stigma for the Self-Esteem of People with Mental Illnesses. *Psychiatric Services*, 52(12): 1621–1626.

Linné, O. and Warfella, E. (1998) In Dickinson, R., Harindranath, R. and Linné, O. (Eds.) *Approaches to Audiences*. London: Arnold.

Lissman, T. and Boehnlein, J. (2001) A Critical Review of Internet Information about Depression. *Psychiatric Services*, 52(8): 1046–1050.

Livingstone, S. (1998) *Making Sense of Television – the Psychology of Audience Inter-pretation* (2nd edn). London: Routledge.

Lothe, J. (2000) *Narrative in Fiction and Film*. Oxford: Oxford University Press.

Lott, T. (1997) *The Scent of Dried Roses*. London: Penguin.

Lowry, M. (1947) *Under the Volcano*. London: Penguin.

Ludwig, A. (1995) *The Price of Greatness: Resolving the Creativity and Madness Controversy*. New York: Guildford Press.

Lukoff, D. (1999) The Mental Health Internet. *Health Care on the Internet*, 3(2): 3–17.

McArdle, S. and Byrt, R. (2001) Fiction, Poetry and Mental Health: Expressive and Therapeutic Uses of Literature. *Journal of Psychiatric and Mental Health Nursing*, 8(6): 517–524.

McCann, R. (2004) *Just a Boy*. London: Ebury Press.

McClure, I. (2000) Driving Mum Crazy. *British Medical Journal*, 320, 388.

McCourt, F. (1996) *Angela's Ashes*. London: Harper Collins.

McDonald, A. and Walter, G. (2001) The Portrayal of ECT in American Movies. *Journal of ECT*, 17(4): 264–274.

McGee, S. and Whitehouse, P. (2005) *Internet Firms Face More Pressure on Suicide Sites*. Available at <http://www.yorkshiretoday.co.uk/ViewArticle2.aspx?

SectionID=55&ArticleID=1218182> (Accessed 4 December 2005).

McGovern, D. and Cope, R. (1987) The Compulsory Detention of Males of Different Ethnic Groups with Special Reference to Offender Patients. *British Journal of Psychiatry*, 150, 505–512.

McGrath, P. (1996) *Asylum*. London: Penguin.

McKenzie, K. (1994) Spot the Loony. *British Medical Journal*, 309, 1588.

McNair, B. (1998) *The Sociology of Journalism*. London: Arnold.

McNair, B. (2003) *News and Journalism in the UK* (4th edn). London: Routledge.

McQuail, D. (1992) *Media Performance: Mass Communication and the Public Interest*. London: Sage.

McQuail, D. (1997) *Audience Analysis*. London: Sage.

McQuail, D. (2000) *McQuail's Mass Communication Theory* (4th edn). London: Sage.

McQuail, D. (2005) McQuail's Mass Communication Theory (5th edn). London: Sage.

McQuail, D. and Windahl, S. (1993) *Communication Models: for the Study of Mass Communications* (2nd edn). London: Longman.

McQuail, D., Blumler, J. and Brown, J. (1972) The Television Audience, a Revised Perspective. In McQuail, D. (ed.) *Sociology of Mass Communication*. Beverly Hills: Sage, pp. 135–164.

Maclennan, G. (1992) *Lucid Interval*. Leicester: Leicester University Press.

Maheu, M. and Barry, G. (2000) Counselling and Therapy on the Internet. *Professional Psychology: Research and Practice*, 31(5): 484–489.

Main, L. (2003) Scare in the Community. *Mental Health Today*. July/August, 8–9.

Manic Depression Fellowship. *MDF the bipolar organisation*. Available at <http://www.mdf.org.uk/bipolar/treatments.html> (Accessed 17 February 2005)

Martin, W. (1986) *Recent Theories of Narrative*. London: Cornell University Press.

Martin, M. and Kennedy, P. (1993) Advertising and Social Comparison: Consequences for Female Preadolescents. *Psychology and Marketing*, 10, 513–530.

Martinez-Gonzalez, M., Gual, P., Lahortiga, F., Alonso, Y., De Irla-Estevez, J. and Cervera, S. (2003) Parental Factors, Mass Media Influences, and the Onset of Eating Disorders in a Prospective Population-Based Cohort. *Pediatrics*, 111(2): 315–320.

Maslow, A. (1971) *The Farther Reaches of Human Nature*. Harmondsworth: Penguin.

Mason, G. (2003) News Media Portrayal of Mental Illness: Implications for Public Policy. *American Behavioural Scientist*, 46(12): 1594–1600.

Mathews, T. (1994) *Censored*. London: Chatto and Windus.

Maurier, D. Du (1992) *Rebecca*. London: Arrow.

Medcircle. *Collaboration for Internet Rating, Certification, Labelling and Evaluation of Health Information*. Available at <www.medcircle.org> (Accessed 12 July 2005).

Media Bureau (2001) *Mental Health and the Press*. Available at <http://www.mhmedia.com/training/report.html. (Accessed 21 July 2005).

Mehlum, L. (2000) Crisis: The Internet, Suicide, and Suicide Prevention. *The Journal of Crisis Intervention and Suicide Prevention*, 21(4): 186–188.

Mental Health Media (2002) *MHM*. Available at www.mhmedia.com (Accessed 21 July 2005).

Mental Health Media (2004) *Mental Health Media's Anti-Discrimination Toolkit*. Available at <http://www.openuptoolkit.net/take_action/the_bill.php> (Accessed 14 July 2005).

Metz, C. (1982) *The Imaginary Signifier: Psychoanalysis and the Cinema*. Bloomington: Indiana University Press.

Miles, A. (1981) *The Mentally Ill in Contemporary Society: a Sociological Introduction*. Oxford: Martin Robertson.

Miller, N. (2002) *But Enough about Me*. New York: Columbia University Press.

Milligan, S. and Clare, A. (1994) *Depression and How to Survive it*. London: Arrow.

Mind (2000) *Counting the Cost: a Survey of the Impact of Media Coverage on the Lives of People with Mental Health Problems*. London: Mind Publications.

Mind (2001) *Mind: for better Mental Health*. Available at <www.mind.org.uk> (Accessed 17 March 2005).

Mind (2004a) *Mind Statement on Draft Mental Health Bill Announcement*. Available at <http://www.mind.org.uk/News+policy+and+campaigns/Press/MHBstate.htm> (Accessed 15 October 2004).

Mind (2004b) *How to Help Someone who is Suicidal*. Available at <www.mind.org.uk> (Accessed 11 July 2005).

Mindout for Mental Health (2001a) *Mindshift: a Guide to Open-Minded Coverage of Mental Health*. Available at <http://mindout.clarity.uk.net/p/mindshift.pdf> (Accessed 11 November 2005).

Mindout for Mental Health (2001b) *Headspace*. Available at <http://www.mindout.net/headspace/lx.asp> (Accessed 20 October 2004).

Mindout for Mental Health (2005) *Mindout for Mental Health*. Available at <http://mindout.clarity.uk.net/iwi/iC2-Camp-info.asp> (Accessed 12 August 2005).

Moore, S. (1988) *Investigating Deviance*. London: Collins Educational.

Moores, S. (1993) *Interpreting Audiences: The Ethnography of Media Consumption*. London: Sage.

Morahan-Martin, J. and Anderson, C. (2000) Information and Misinformation Online: Recommendations for Facilitating Accurate Mental Health Information Retrieval and Evaluation. *Cyberpsychology and Behaviour*, 3(5): 731–746.

Mori (2001) *Mori Poll: Nearly 3 out of 5 Internet Users Would Seek Help for Mental Health Problems on the Net*. Available at <www.mori.com/polls/2001/zeus.shtml> (Accessed 22 July 2005).

Morrall, P. (2000a) *Madness and Murder*. London: Whurr.

Morrall, P. (2000b) Madness and Murder. *Mental Health Practice*, 4(1): 8–10.

Motion Picture Association of America (2003) *Motion Picture Association of America*. Available at <http://mpaa.org/about/content.htm> (Accessed 27 November 2003).

Murdock, G. (1998) Mass Communication and the Construction of Meaning. In Dickinson, R., Harindranath, R. and Linné, O. (eds) *Approaches to Audiences*. London: Arnold, pp. 205–217.

Myers, P. and Biocca, F. (1992) The Elastic Body Image: the Effect of Television Advertising and Programming on Body Image Distortion in Young Women. *Journal of Communication*, 42 (3): 108–133.

Nairn, R., Coverdale, J. and Claasen, D. (2001) From Source Material to News Story in New Zealand Print Media: a Prospective Study of the Stigmatising Processes in Depicting Mental Illness. *Australian and New Zealand Journal of Psychiatry*, 35, 654–659.

Nasar, S. (1998) *A Beautiful Mind*. London: Faber and Faber.

National Patient Safety Agency (2001) Safety First, National Confidential Inquiry into Suicide and Homicide by People with Mental Illness, five-year report of the National Confidential Inquiry.

National Union of Journalists (1999) *Code of Conduct*. Available at <http://www.nuj.org.uk/inner.php?docid=59> (Accessed 12 July 2005).

National Union of Journalists/Royal College of Psychiatry (1999) *Guide for Journalists and Broadcasters Reporting on Schizophrenia*. Dublin: Lilly Neuroscience Bureau.

Nelson, R. (1997) *TV Drama in Transition – Forms, Values and Cultural Change.* London: Macmillan.

Nettle, D. (2001) *Strong Imagination: Madness Creativity and Human Nature.* Oxford: Oxford University Press.

Nimmo, D. and Combs, J. (1983) *Mediated Political Realities.* New York: Longman.

Noble, G. (1973) Effects of Different Forms of Filmed Aggression on Children's Constructive and Deconstructive Play. *Journal of Personality and Social Psychology,* 26, 54–59.

Norden, M. (1994) *The Cinema of Isolation.* New Jersey: Rutgers University Press.

Nunnally, J. (1981) Mental Illness: What the Media Present. In Cohen, S. and Young, J. (eds) *The Manufacture of News: Deviance, Social Problems and the Mass Media.* Beverly Hills: Sage, pp. 186–196.

O'Connor, J. and Seymour, J. (1990) *Introducing Neurolinguistic Programming. Psychological Skills for Understanding and Influencing People.* London: Aquarian.

Ofcom. *Office of Communications.* Available at <www.ofcom.org.uk> (Accessed 14 June 2005).

Ofcom. (2004) *The Ofcom Internet and Broadband Update.* Available at <http://www.ofcom.org.uk/research/telecoms/reports/bbresearch/int_bband_updt/may2004/#content> (Accessed 24 November 2005).

Ofcom (2005) *Ofcom Broadcasting Code.* Available at <http://www.ofcom.org.uk/tv/ifi/codes/bcode/ofcom-broadcasting-code.pdf> (Accessed 6 December 2005).

O'Gunleye, I. (2003) My Descent into Psychosis. *The Independent on Sunday,* 26 October, pp. 1–2.

Oravec, J. (2000) Online Counselling and the Internet: Perspectives for Mental Health Care Supervision and Education. *Journal of Mental Health,* 9(2): 121–135.

Östman, M. and Kjellin, L. (2002) Stigma by Association. Psychological Factors in Relatives of People with Mental Illness. *British Journal of Psychiatry,* 181, 494–498.

O'Sullivan, T., Dutton, B. and Rayner, P. (1994) *Studying the Media: An Introduction.* London: Arnold.

Oxford English Dictionary (2005) Available at <www.oed.com> (Acccessed 19 July 2005)

Padel, R. (1995) *Whom Gods Destroy.* Princeton NJ: Princeton University Press.

Paletz, D. and Entman, R. (1981) *Media, Power, Politics.* New York: Free Press.

Palmgreen, P. and Rayburn, J. (1985) An Expectancy-Value approach to Media Gratification. In Rosengren, K., Palmgreen, P. and Wenner, L. (eds) *Media Gratification Research: Current Perspectives.* Beverly Hills: Sage, pp. 61–73.

Pasternak, B. (1978) *Doctor Zhivago.* London: Collins.

Pavlov, I. (1958) *Experimental Psychology and Other Essays.* London: Peter Owen.

Pegler, J. (2003) Mad Memoirs of the 21st Century. *Mental Health Today,* November, 31–33.

Pelzer, D. (1995) *A Child Called It.* London: Orion.

Pelzer, D. (1997) *The Lost Boy.* London: Orion.

Pelzer, D. (1999) *A Man Named Dave.* London: Orion.

Pelzer, D. (2004) *My Story.* London: Orion.

Pelzer, D. (2005) *The Privilege of Youth.* London: Penguin.

Pelzer, R. (2005) *A Brother's Journey.* London: Time Warner.

Penn, D., Guynan, K., Daily, T., Spaulding, W., Garbin, C. and Sullivan, M. (1994) Dispelling the Stigma of Schizophrenia: What sort of Information is Best? *Schizophrenia Bulletin,* 20(3): 567–574.

Penny, J. (1992) *I Have What I Gave: the Fiction of Janet Frame*. Wellington: Daphne Brassell Associates Press.

Peplau, H. (1988) *Interpersonal Relations in Nursing: a Conceptual Frame of Reference for Psychodynamic Nursing*. Basingstoke: Macmillan Education.

Persaud, R. (2000) Psychiatrists Suffer from Stigma too. *Psychiatric Bulletin*, 24, 284–285.

Peters, C. (2002) Doctor's Bad Press Depends on Type of Newspaper. *British Medical Journal*, 324, 241.

Petley, J. (1999) The Regulation of Media Content. In Stokes, J. and Reading, A. (eds) *The Media in Britain*. New York: St Martin's Press, pp. 143–157.

Petty, R. and Priester, J. (1994) Mass Media Attitude Change: Implications of the Elaboration Likelihood Model of Persuasion. In Bryant, J. and Zillman, D. (eds) *Media Effects: Advances in Theory and Research*. New Jersey: Lawrence Erlbaum, pp. 91–122.

Philo, G. (1990) *Seeing is Believing: The Influence of Television*. London: Routledge.

Philo, G. (1996a) The Media and Public Belief. In Philo, G. (ed.) *Media and Mental Distress*. London: Longman, pp. 82–104.

Philo, G. (1996b) Introduction. In Philo, G. (ed.) *Media and Mental Distress*. London: Longman, pp. xi–xv

Philo, G. (1996c) Users of Services, Carers and Families. In Philo, G. (ed.) *Media and Mental Distress*. London: Longman, pp. 105–118.

Philo, G. (1999) Media and Mental Illness. In Philo, G. (ed.) *Message Received*. Harlow: Addison Wesley Longman, pp. 54–61.

Philo, G., McLaughlin, G. and Henderson, L. (1996) Media Content. In Philo, G. (ed.) *Media and Mental Distress*. London: Longman, pp. 45–81.

Philo, G., Secker, J. and Platts, S. (1994) Impact of the Mass Media on Public Images of Mental Illness: Media Content and Audience Belief. *Health Education Journal*, 53, 271–281.

Piaget, J. (1958) *The Growth of Logical Thinking from Childhood to Adolescence*. London: Routledge.

Piercy, M. (1976) *Woman on the Edge of Time*. London: The Women's Press.

Pinfold, V. (2003) Awareness in Action. *Mental Health Today*, July/August, 24–25.

Pirkis, J. and Blood, R. (2001) Suicide and the Media: Part II: Portrayal in Fictional Media. *Crisis: The Journal of Crisis Intervention and Suicide Prevention*, 22(4): 155–162.

Plath, S. (1963) *The Bell Jar*. London: Faber and Faber.

Porter, R. (2002) *Madness: a Brief History*. Oxford: Oxford University Press.

Post, F. (1994) Creativity and Psychopathology: A Study of 291 World-Famous Men. *British Journal of Psychiatry*, 164, 22–34.

Potter, W. (1998) *Media Literacy*. London: Sage

Potter, W. (2004) *Theory of Media Literacy: a Cognitive Approach*. London: Sage.

Powell, J. and Clarke, A. (2002) The www of the World Wide Web: Who What and Why.? *Journal of Medical Internet Resources*, 4: E4 ⊏medline⊐.

Prendergast, R. (1992) *Film Music: a Neglected Art: a Critical Study of Music in Films* (2nd edn). London: Norton.

Press Complaints Commission (2000) *Past Decisions*. Available at <http://www.pcc.org.uk/reports/details.asp?id=56> (Accessed 18 July 2005).

Press Complaints Commission. (2005) *Code of Practice*. Available at <http://www.pcc.org.uk/cop/cop.asp> (Accessed 12 July 2005).

Priebe, S. (2003) Media Coverage of Mental Health Care in the UK, USA and Australia. *Psychiatric Bulletin*, 27, 331–333.

Prior, C. (2003) *Shocked Sun readers show national anti-stigma campaign needed.* Available at <http://www.rethink.org/news%2Bcampaigns/press_releases/frank-bruno.htm> (Accessed 24 September 2003).

Pursehouse, M. (1991) Looking at *The Sun*: into the Nineties with a Tabloid and its Readers. *Cultural Studies at Birmingham*, 1, 88–133.

Repper, J., Sayce, L., Strong, S., Wilmot, J. and Haines, M. (1997) *Tall Stories from the Backyard*. London: Mind.

Ressler, R. and Schachtman, T. (1992) *Whoever Fights Monsters*. New York: St Martin's Press.

Rethink (2002) *Severe Mental Illness*. Available at <www.rethink.org> (Accessed 20 May 2005).

Rethink (2004) *Severe Mental Illness*. Available at <http://www.rethink.org/> (Accessed 15 November 2004).

Riddell, M. (2002) The Fiction of New Fiction. *Observer Sunday*, 22 September.

Robinson, J. and Levy, M. (1986) *The Main Source*. London: Sage.

Roediger, H., Rushton, J., Capaldi, E. and Paris, S. (1991) *Psychology* (3rd edn). New York: HarperCollins.

Rogers, C. (1951) *Client Centred Therapy: its Current Practice, Implications and Theory*. London: Constable.

Rogers, C. (1961) *On Becoming a Person: a Therapist's View of Psychotherapy*. Boston: Houghton Mifflin.

Rogers, E. (1986) *Communication Technology*. New York: Free Press.

Rogers, A., Pilgrim, D. and Lacey, R. (1993) *Experiencing Psychiatry: User's Views of Services*. London: Macmillan.

Rosen, A. and Walter, G. (2000) Way out of Tune: Lessons from Shine and its Expose. *Australian and New Zealand Journal of Psychiatry*, 34, 237–244.

Rosengren, K. and Windahl, S. (1989) *Media Matter: TV use in Childhood and Adolescence*. Norwood NJ: Ablex.

Rosenhan, D. (1973) On Being Sane in Insane Places. *Science*, 179, 250–258.

Rothbart, M. and Park, B. (1986) On the Confirmability and Disconfirmability of Trait Concepts. *Journal of Personality and Social Psychology*, 50, 131–142.

Rothbart, M., Fulero, S. and Jensen, C. (1978) From Individual to Group Impressions: Availability Heuristics in Stereotype Formation. *Journal of Experimental Social Psychology*, 14, 237–255.

Rothman, W. (1988) *The 'I' of the Camera: Essays in Film Criticism, History and Aesthetics*. Cambridge: Cambridge University Press.

Rowling, J. K. (2000) *Harry Potter and the Goblet of Fire*. London: Bloomsbury.

Royal College of Psychiatrists (2001) *Changing Minds: Every Family in the Land*. Available at http://www.stigma.org/everyfamily/everycontentsnew.html (Accessed 21 July 2005).

Royal College of Psychiatrists (2005) *2001: A Mind Odyssey*. Available at http://www.rcpsych.ac.uk/campaigns/2001/ (Accessed at 18 June 2005).

Rubin, A. (1984) Ritualised and Instrumental Television Viewing. *Journal of Communication*, 34(3): 67–77.

Rushdie, S. (1994) *The Satanic Verses*. London: Vintage.

Salkeld, D. (1993) *Madness and Drama in the Age of Shakespeare*. Manchester: Manchester University Press.

Salter, M. (2003) Psychiatry and the Media: from Pitfalls to Possibilities. *Psychiatric Bulletin*, 27, 123–125.

Salter, M. and Byrne, P. (2000) The Stigma of Mental Illness: How You can Use the Media to Reduce it. *Psychiatric Bulletin*, 24, 281–283.

Samaritans (1997) *Media Guidelines on Portrayals of Suicide*. Online booklet, Available at <www.samaritans.org.uk> (Accessed 12 July 2005).

Samaritans (2005) *Samaritans*. Available at <http://www.samaritans.org.uk/> (Accessed 22 July 2005).

SANE (2003) *SANE*. Available at http://www.sane.org.uk/ (Accessed 24 September 2003).

Sartorius, N. (2002) Iatrogenic Stigma of Mental Illness: Begins with Behaviour and Attitudes of Medical Professionals, Especially Psychiatrists. *British Medical Journal*, 324(7352): 1470–1471.

Sartre, J. P. (1967) *What is Literature*. London: Methuen.

Say No To Psychiatry. *Say No To Psychiatry*. Available at <http://www.sntp.net/> (Accessed 12 May 2005).

Sayce, L. (2000) *From Psychiatric Patient to Citizen*. London: Macmillan.

Scambler, G. (1998) Stigma and Disease: Changing Paradigms. *Lancet*, 352, 1054–1055.

Scheff, T. (1968) The Role of the Mentally Ill and the Dynamics of Mental Disorder. In Spitzer, S. and Denzin, N. *The Mental Patient*. London: McGraw Hill, pp. 8–22.

Scheff, T. (1974) The Labelling Theory of Mental Illness. *American Sociological Review*, 39, 444–452.

Schlesinger, J. (2002a) Issues in Creativity and Madness Part One: Ancient Questions, Modern Answers. *Ethical Human Sciences & Services*, 4(1): 73–76.

Schlesinger, J. (2002b) Issues in Creativity and Madness Part Two: Eternal Flames. *Ethical Human Sciences & Services*, 4(2): 139–142.

Schmidtke, A. and Schaller, S. (2000) The Role of Mass Media in Suicide Prevention. In Hawton, K. and van Heeringen, K. (eds) *The International Handbook of Suicide and Attempted Suicide*. New York: Wiley, pp. 675–697.

Schneider, I. (1987) The Theory and Practice of Movie Psychiatry. *American Journal of Psychiatry*, 144(8): 996–1002.

Scrivener, R. (2002) *Mapping Health on the Internet*. Abingdon: Radcliffe Medical Press.

Seale, C. (2002) *Media and Health*. London: Sage.

Secker, J. and Platt, S. (1996) Why Media Images Matter. In Philo, G. (ed.) *Media and Mental Distress*. London: Longman, pp. 1–17.

Sen, D. (2003) Mad Memoirs of the 21st Century. *Mental Health Today*, November, pp. 31–33.

Serenity. Available at <http://www.findserenitynow.com/uk/index.html> (Accessed 29 April 2005).

Shakespeare, W. (1972) *King Lear* (9th edn). London: Methuen.

Sheldon, T. (1996) Public Therapy. *British Medical Journal*, 313, 238 (27 July).

Shelley, M. (1818) *Frankenstein*. London: Penguin.

Shoemaker, P. and Reese, S. (1996) *Mediating the Message: Theories of Influences on Mass Media Content* (2nd edn). London: Longman.

Shore, B. (1996) *Culture in Mind. Cognition, Culture and the Problem of Meaning*. New York: Oxford University Press.

Sieff, E. (2003) Media Frames of Mental Illnesses: The Potential Impact of Negative Frames. *Journal of Mental Health*, 12(3): 259–269.

Signorielli, N. (1989) The Stigma of Mental Illness on Television. *Journal of Broadcasting and Electronic Media*, 33(3): 325–31.

Simon, B. (1978) *Mind and Madness in Ancient Greece. The Classical Roots of Modern Psychiatry*. London: Cornell University Press.

Skinner, B. (1974) *About Behaviourism*. New York: Alfred Knopf.

Skynner, R. and Cleese, J. (1993) *Families and How to Survive Them*. London: Mandarin.

Slattery, K., Doremus, M. and Marcus, L. (2001) Shifts in Public Affairs Reporting on the Network Evening News: A Move to the Sensational. *Journal of Broadcasting and Electronic Media*, 45, 290–292.

Small, H. (1996) *Love's Madness. Medicine, the Novel and Female Insanity 1800–1865*. Oxford: Clarendon Press.

Smith, M. (2002) Stigma. *Advances in Psychiatric Treatment*, 8, 317–325.

Snoddy, R. (1993) *The Good, The Bad and the Unacceptable*. London: Faber and Faber.

Social Exclusion Unit (2003) *Mental Health and Social Exclusion. Consultation Document*. Available at <http://www.socialexclusionunit.gov.uk/downloaddoc.asp?id=44> (Accessed 20 July 2005).

Solomon, A. (2002) *The Noonday Demon: an Anatomy of Depression*. London: Vintage.

Solzhenitsyn, I. (1963) *One Day in the Life of Ivan Denisovich*. London: Penguin.

Solzhenitsyn, I. (1974) *The Gulag Archipelago*. New York: Viking.

Squires, J. (1993) *Read all about it! The Corporate Takeover of America's Newspapers*. New York: Times Books.

Stevenson, N. (2002) *Understanding Media Cultures* (2nd edn). London: Sage.

Stice, E. and Shaw, H. (1994) Adverse Effects of the Media Portrayed Thin-Ideal on Women, and Linkages to Bulimic Symptoms. *Journal of Social and Clinical Psychology*, 13, 288–305.

Susman, J. (1994) Disability, Stigma and Deviance. *Social Science & Medicine*, 38(1): 15–22.

Szasz, T. (1992) The Myth of Mental Illness. In Miller, R. (ed.) *The Restoration of Dialogue: Readings in the Philosophy of Clinical Psychology*. Washington: American Psychological Association, pp.175–182.

Tam, P. (2002) Psychiatry and the Cinema. *Australasian Psychiatry*, 10(2): 178.

Taylor, P. and Gunn, J. (1999) Homicides by People with Mental Illness: Myth and Reality. *British Journal of Psychiatry*, 174, 9–14.

Thede, L. (1999) *Computers in Nursing*. New York: Lippincott.

Thompson, S. (1999) The Internet and its Potential Influence on Suicide. *Psychiatric Bulletin*, 23 (8): 449–451.

Tomaiuolo, N. (1995) Accessing Nursing Resources on the Internet. *Computers in Nursing*, 13(4): 159–164.

Turner, G. (1999) *Film as Social Practice* (3rd edn). London: Routledge.

Unsworth, J. (1995) Why Does an Author who Apparently Draws so Much on Autobiography seem Committed to Alienating the Reader? In Swindells, J. (ed.) *The Uses of Autobiography*. London: Taylor & Francis, pp. 24–29.

Valenti, M. (2000) *More than a Movie: Ethics in Entertainment*. Oxford: Westview Press.

Van Dijk, T. (1987) *Communicating Racism: Ethnic Prejudice in Thought and Talk*. Newbury Park: Sage.

Vedic Wisdom. *Vedic Wisdom*. Available at <http://www.vedicwisdom.com/decure.html> (Accessed 24 June 2005).

Von Goethe, J. (1989) [1774]. *The Sorrows of Young Werther*. Trans Michael Hulse. London: Penguin.

Vooijs, M. and Van der Voort, T. (1993) Learning about Television Violence: the Impact of a Critical Viewing Curriculum on Children's Attitudinal Judgements of Crime Series. *Journal of Research and Development in Education*, 26(3): 133–142

Vousden, M. (1989) 'Loony Lefties' and 'Mad Mullahs'. *Nursing Times*, 85(28): 16–17.

Waddell, C. (1998) Creativity and Mental illness: Is there a Link? *Canadian Journal of Psychiatry*, 43(2): 166–172.

Wahl, O. (1995) *Media Madness: Public Images of Mental Illness*. New Brunswick, NJ: Rutgers University Press.

Wahl, O., Wood, A. and Richards, R. (2002) Newspaper Coverage of Mental Illness: Is it Changing? *Psychiatric Rehabilitation Skills*, 6(1): 9–31.

Wahl, O. (2003a) Depictions of Mental Illness in Children's Media. *Journal of Mental Health*, 12(3): 249–258.

Wahl, O. (2003b) News Media Portrayal of Mental Illness: Implications for Public Policy. *American Behavioural Scientist*, 46(12): 1594–1600.

Wahl, O. and Kaye, A. (1992) Mental Illness Topics in Popular Periodicals. *Community Mental Health Journal*, 28(1): 21–28.

Wall, B. and Rossen, E. (2004) Media as a Teaching Tool in Psychiatric Nursing Education. *Nurse Educator*, 29(1): 36–40.

Walsh, A. (2002) *E-Mail Correspondence*. Channel 4 Disability Advisor. 5th June 2002.

Wedding, D. and Boyd, M. (1999) *Movies and Mental Illness*. Boston, MA: McGraw Hill Education.

Weiss, M., Sushrut, J., Raguram, R., Vounatsou, P. and Littlewood, R. (2001) Psychiatric Stigma across Cultures: Local Validation in Bangalore and London. *Anthropology and Medicine*, 8(1): 71–87.

Welch, M. and Racine, T. (1999) A Psycho for Every Generation. *Nursing Inquiry*, 6(3): 216–219.

White, R. (1990) The Birth of the Reader. In McGregor, G. and White, R. (eds) *Reception and Response – Hearer Creativity and the Analysis of Spoken and Written Texts*. London: Routledge, pp. 242–259.

Williams, M. and Taylor, J. (1995) Mental Illness: Media Perpetuation of Stigma. *Contemporary Nurse*, 4(1): 41–46.

Williams, R. (2002) *Somebody Someday*. London: Ebury Press.

Wilson, C., Nairn, R., Coverdale, J. and Panapa, A. (1999) Mental Illness Depictions in Prime-Time Drama: Identifying the Discursive Resources. *Australian and New Zealand Journal of Psychiatry*, 33, 232–239.

Wilson, C., Nairn, R., Coverdale, J. and Panapa, A. (2000) How Mental Illness is Portrayed in Children's Television. *British Journal of Psychiatry*, 176, 440–443.

Wilson, M. (1997) Printing it in Black and White. *OpenMind*, 85, May/June, 16–17.

Wing, J. (1978) *Reasoning about Madness*. Oxford: Oxford University Press.

Winker, M., Flanagin, A., Chi-Lum, B., White, J., Andrews, K., Kennett, R., DeAngelis, C. and Musacchio, R. (2000) Guidelines for Medical and Health Information Sites on the Internet: Principles Governing AMA Web Sites. *Journal of the American Medical Association*, 283(12): 1600–1606.

Winship, J. (1987) *Inside Women's Magazines*. London: Pandora.

Wober, J. (1991) *Television and Mental Ill Health*. London: Independent Television Commission Research Monographs.

Wolfenstein, M. and Leites, N. (1970) *Movies: A Psychological Study* (2nd edn). New York: Atheneum.

Woods, R. (2002) The Death of Dignity. *Sunday Times*, 21 July.

Woolf, L. (ed.) (1953) *A Writer's Diary: Virginia Woolf*. London: Hogarth Press.

World Federation for Mental Health (2005) *World Mental Health Day*. Available at <http://www.wfmh.org/wmhday2005.htm> (Accessed 6 December 2005).

Wright, T. (1997) Creativity and Bipolar Disorder. *Medical Problems of Performing Artists*, 12(3): 89–92.

Wurtzel, E. (1994) *Prozac Nation*. London: Quartet Books.

Wykes, M. and Gunter, B. (2005) *The Media and Body Image*. London: Sage.

Yalom, I. (1995) *The Theory and Practice of Group Psychotherapy* (4th edn). New York: Basic Books.

Ying, H. (1999) *Daughter of the River*. London: Bloomsbury.

Young, R. (1991) Poems that Read Themselves. *Tropismes*, 5, 233–261.

Zillmann, D. (1980) Anatomy of Suspense. In Tannebaum, P. (ed.) *The Entertainment Functions of Television*. New Jersey: Lawrence Erlbaum.

Zito Trust (2005) *The Zito Trust*. Available at <http://www.zitotrust.co.uk/> (Accessed 12 July 2005).

Index

Lightning Source UK Ltd.
Milton Keynes UK
UKOW06f0124241115

263390UK00003B/57/P